The
Other Side
of
Pregnancy

The Other Side of Pregnancy

A Doctor and Dad Looks at Reducing Neck and Back Pain During and After Pregnancy

Trenton L. Scott D.C., L.Ac
with Rick Sawyer

To order additional copies of this book, contact:
Xlibris Corporation
1-888-795-4274
www.Xlibris.com
Orders@Xlibris.com
46781

"Great book! It is interesting and very entertaining"

Stephanie Simmonds RN

Mother of 3

"Dr. Scott has compiled a great amount of knowledge in an entertaining and accessible book!"

"This book is a must have for anyone wishing to have a healthy and pain free pregnancy."

Michah Stephens L.Ac, M.S.O.M

"Dr. Scott clarifies the benefits of alternative health care and in our busy world gives practical advice on how to help yourself when you are in pain."

Jahna Brazier, CMT

"If you've ever had back trouble then you know the importance of keeping it healthy!" Dr. Scott's book is a wonderful preventative resource for all mothers. His wisdom is invaluable for the health of your back."

Heather hill

Mother of 3

Littleton, CO

CONTENTS

SECTION 3: YOUR BABY'S BIG DAY

SECTION 4: AFTER YOU'VE GIVEN BIRTH

DEDICATION

This book is dedicated to my wife; mother and all my patients that have let me help them bring a life into this world.

Dr. Trenton Scott D.C., L.Ac

PREFACE

I've read many books and visited numerous Web sites on pregnancy over the past several years. More than a few do such a great job of alarming the reader about the various maladies, troubles, and conditions that can develop during that very special nine-month period that even *I* thought I had a problem pregnancy.

Fortunately, my wife reminded me that I was ill equipped. It turns out I was just a little chunky and had eaten some bad bean dip.

All kidding aside, in writing this book, it was not our intention to frighten or worry you. Please don't read this book and diagnose your condition based on just this information. The point of this book is to empower expectant mothers and to give each of you some insight that you might not get elsewhere on the causes and treatments for neck and back pain before and after the birth of your baby.

Hopefully, this book will do more than simply help you cope with back pain associated with pregnancy. Our goal is to dramatically decrease back pain, relieve back pain, and even, in some cases, eliminate back pain.

It's not acceptable for me to just say to a mom-to-be, "Okay, you have back pain. So does every other woman in your condition. Tough it out."

No way! It's *not* okay! I work with patients every day to relieve neck pain, lower-back pain, and headaches. My practice has attracted a great number of pregnant women, so I know you don't have to accept those conditions as "normal."

Usually, it's the women who've come to me as a last-ditch effort for their neck or back pain that have become my biggest fans. I quickly go from their last resort to their hero. It is common to hear, "I wish I would have seen you sooner!"

So do I.

So when you're reading this book, please strive to be open-minded. Allow my experience to give you ideas, knowledge, and understanding; and then consult with your obstetrician or midwife.

You are pregnant, and we don't need you getting stressed or paranoid in any way while reading this book. I wrote this so you can better enjoy the excitement of bringing a new life into this world.

INTRODUCTION

Welcome to the other side of childbirth, the back side. While the miracle of life is growing in front of you, at least one out of every two expectant or new moms is experiencing backache, sometimes severe, debilitating back pain.

The bad news is that even if this is your second or third child on the way and you never endured back pain before, you may well experience it this time.

In fact, each successive pregnancy weakens the ligaments supporting your spinal column, so the chances of back pain actually increase with each subsequent child.

Also complicating the process is that some women who don't experience back pain during their pregnancy develop back pain either during labor or after the baby is born.

The good news is that there are things you can do to make back pain virtually a nonissue throughout your pregnancy experience. It isn't always easy, and it will take some effort on your part; but most pregnancy-related back pain is avoidable or, at the very least, manageable.

How can I be so confident? It's my job. I've worked with hundreds of pregnant women, and I have more than a decade of clinical experience with moms-to-be.

I have a thriving chiropractic practice in Loveland, Colorado, that I started well over a decade ago with my lovely wife, Gina, who is also a doctor of chiropractic. Gina and I have four beautiful children, so we have ample firsthand knowledge of the challenges your back is facing with your pregnancy.

Gina claims I became an expert on eliminating back pain in pregnancy because I felt guilty for causing her discomfort.

She knows me too well.

Many women don't even consider chiropractic treatment for back pain during pregnancy until they reach a point of intense, unrelenting discomfort. In my business, pain is a proven motivator. I regularly see pregnant women in distress.

When ladies finally come into the office to see me, I'm usually able to help them. This book contains some of the things I've learned, some of the tactics I've used, and some stories of the women I've helped. Hopefully, by reading this, I can help you too.

After you read this book, I'm confident that you'll seriously consider adding a doctor of chiropractic with special knowledge related to back pain in pregnancy to your health care team. You'll soon learn that I believe you need a team of qualified health care professionals to achieve a pain-free pregnancy.

Your pregnancy is the miracle of life, and you should enjoy it without the distraction of back pain.

What can a man tell a woman about being pregnant?

It's okay to admit it. That's what you might have been thinking.

Obviously, I have never, as Lily Tomlin put it so eloquently, "pulled my lower lip over my head." I have not had my nipples get so sensitive I wanted to cry nor has my skin stretched so tightly around my belly that I feel like a ripe cantaloupe. I've also never been forced to shuffle around like a penguin.

What I have done, though, is suffer from back pain. I currently have disc herniation over the lumbar spine. I won't bore you with my medical history, just suffice it to say that I have experienced debilitating back pain firsthand.

And I know neck and back pain from a clinical perspective. I have been treating pregnant women since some of my current pregnant patients were still in grade school.

I have also treated and coached my wife through the births of our four children.

Wow, a coach . . .

I sense some skepticism out there. Hey, don't knock my position as a coach. It takes a different skill set to perform than it does to coach. The best players are very rarely the best coaches. The fact that I can't give birth is a terrific qualification for being a coach. It's a historical reality. Look it up.

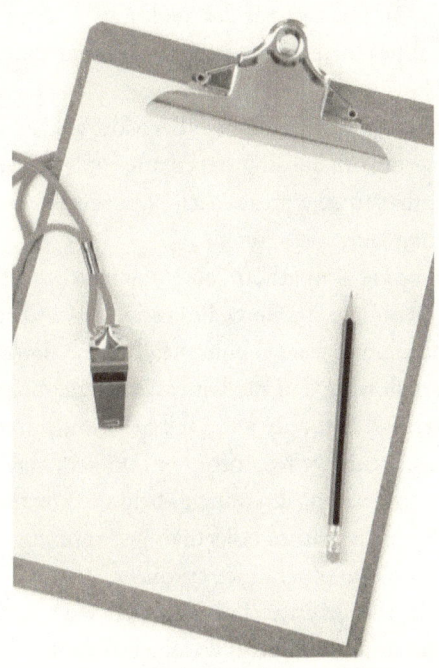

I'm a sports fan. In fact, I'm the chiropractor on the sports medicine staffs of both our local professional hockey team and our indoor football team. One thing I know about coaching is that the superstar coaches are usually guys who never stood out on the highest level as competitors. Great coaches are generally the players who spent their careers sitting on the bench or, at best, were classified as *role players*. Very few athletes who became household names have ever excelled as coaches.

For example, Vince Lombardi, a pro football coaching icon, played college football but was never a player on a professional team.

Baseball Hall of Fame manager Tommy Lasorda was a star minor-league pitcher (the Montreal Royals of the International League) but never established himself as a major-league-caliber player.

As a professional football player, Don Shula was a defensive back drafted in the ninth round in 1951. He played for three teams for over six seasons. He *coached* in the National Football League for thirty-three seasons. He holds records for regular-season wins, total victories, single-season winning percentage (his Miami Dolphins won every game they played in 1972), most games coached, most consecutive seasons coached, and most Super Bowl appearances. He wasn't a superstar player, but he was a truly terrific coach.

On the other side of the coin, three-time NBA Most Valuable Player Magic Johnson quit coaching in frustration with a losing record after only eleven games.

The bottom line is that to be a great coach, you need to be a keen, well-schooled observer, not a star participant.

I consider myself a very empathetic and objective coach in helping my wife understand what is happening to her body. Professional *doulas* (the current movement toward labor support personnel; see *doulas* in the glossary) don't have anything on me!

When hormones are flowing and my wife asks me six different times in an hour, "Why is my back is hurting?" not only will I tell her calmly and compassionately, but I'll treat her back and neck, rub her feet, tuck her into bed, and read her a story.

My point is: men in love will do anything to help their mate out of trouble or pain. We are actually useful for more critical tasks than just running to the grocery store for a jar of pickles and a tub of butter pecan ice cream.

As I've explained, in my practice, I've answered years of questions and treated hundreds of mothers and mothers-to-be. It was the lack of information available on the market today that prompted this book. If you think about it, I'm already one of your coaches by virtue of the information in this book.

My hope is this book can help thousands of mothers that I might otherwise not get to meet. And as your coach, I recommend that you let the man in your life read parts of this book. Perhaps my next book should focus on teaching expectant dads to become great coaches.

SECTION 1

YOUR NEW CHALLENGE

CHAPTER 1

YOUR PREGNANCY

What's going on with my body?

I'll go into greater detail about your back throughout the rest of the book. Let's set the stage, though, with a quick review of your pregnancy in general terms.

Pregnancy 101 Basics

Congratulations on the miracle that's happening inside your body. As a man, I miss out on the wonder of a new life growing inside of me. And that's probably a good thing because pregnancy isn't for wimps, and there is absolutely no evidence that humans of the male persuasion could handle the trauma.

Before we get into specifics, you need to understand some basic health issues related to pregnancy. First of all, pregnancy is a normal, healthy condition for women. It's a wonderful experience. (Or so I've been told.) But you need to be aware that your body is going to go through a great many changes.

First of all, pregnancy is a normal, healthy condition for women. It's a wonderful experience. (Or so I've been told.)

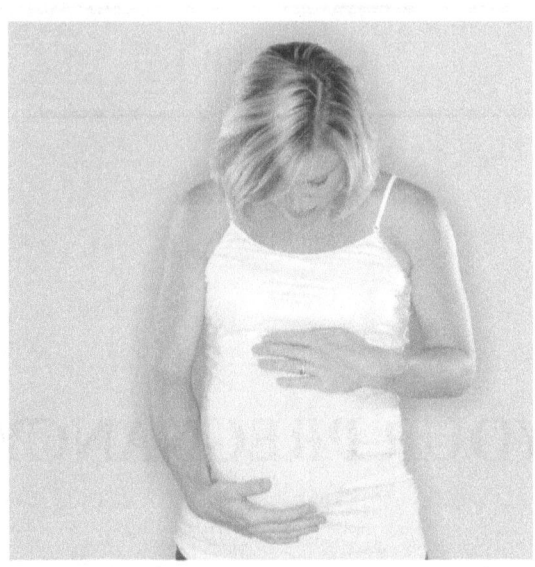

Since your pregnancy is nine months long, we refer to it in three-month increments: the first three months we call the *first trimester*, the fourth through sixth months we refer to as the *second trimester*, and the final three months are the *third trimester*.

During the first trimester, the different parts of the baby are formed. That's when the baby is at greatest risk for harm. In the second and third trimesters, the baby's organs develop and mature, and his or her size and weight increase. (And so do yours!)

Hormones

Your body's changes during pregnancy are caused by chemical messengers that we call *hormones*. There are a few notable hormones involved in pregnancy—*progesterone*, *estrogen*, and others including *relaxin*.

The good-news-bad-news hormone is progesterone. It not only relaxes the muscles of your uterus, where your baby is developing, as well as your stomach and blood vessels, it can also cause some unwanted side effects like indigestion, constipation, heartburn, and varicose veins.

Estrogen plays an important role in your baby's growth and your own breast development.

As far as back pain is concerned, the hormone relaxin causes your ligaments to loosen to get ready for the baby's growth and delivery, making your muscles do extra work to compensate.

Muscles, Joints, and Ligaments

Throughout your pregnancy, the muscles and ligaments of your pelvis relax, softening and stretching to increase the size of your pelvis to accommodate your baby.

Several joints, especially in your spine, will also become less stable and show signs of separation and movement to make room for your growing little darling.

Because the joints in your back become less effective and your ligaments, which are intended to add support and strength, are weakened hormonally, your back muscles need to work harder than ever before. These muscles experience unaccustomed strain, causing some of the low-back pain you may already be suffering.

All of this is explained in greater detail in the appendices in the back of this book.

CHAPTER 2

YOUR BACK

Why am I concerned about my back?

We never think about our back until it starts hurting. But throughout your life, your lower back is the hardest-working part of your body. First of all, it bears two-thirds of your body weight when you're doing any activity other than lying down. Secondly, your legs, rib cage, and head are all attached to your spinal column; so your back is integrally involved in all of your body's movements.

Think about that for a moment: your lower back supports all of the weight above your hips sixteen or more hours a day, every day of your life. If you weigh 120 pounds, your back supports eighty pounds whenever you're not asleep. No other structure in your body was designed to carry that great a load continually, day in and day out, every minute you're awake for your entire life.

Back pain in any form at any time of life causes tremendous physical, mental, and emotional exhaustion. The back is simply too vital to the core of the human body to not cause major complications when it fails to function properly.

How do you know your back isn't functioning the way it was designed? It tells you with pain.

In some cases, lots of pain.

A nagging backache can disrupt your daily routine and interfere with a good night's sleep. Back pain is one of the most common complaints heard in the medical community today.

And statistically, we know that at least one out of every two pregnant women suffers back pain either during pregnancy or after. If that sounds like an enormous number, it's probably quite conservative. I've seen statistics that suggest as many as 70 to 80 percent of pregnant American women suffer back pain during pregnancy. Back pain in this day and age is so prevalent, it's almost always expected to rear its ugly head during your pregnancy.

Although back pain is expected, there's no reason for it to be accepted.

Although back pain is expected, there's no reason for it to be accepted.

Back pain is a common complaint during pregnancy, but it isn't *normal.* The fact that more than 50 percent of women will suffer back pain while pregnant is an unfortunate statistic because back pain is mostly avoidable and, at worst, manageable.

With pregnant women, back pain occurs most frequently in the later months as the weight of the baby increases. In my practice, though, I have treated women who have experienced back pain at every point along the way during their pregnancy and after.

I'm not going to shock you by reminding you that you'll be adding twenty to thirty pounds of concentrated, asymmetrical, sometimes wriggling weight in a place and position that's unusual for your body.

That little bundle of joy growing in your tummy will invariably put new demands on your back.

Back pain is a common complaint during pregnancy, but it isn't normal.

NOT ALL OB-GYNS ARE ENLIGHTENED

I once had a patient we'll call Margie. Margie had been coming to me for several years for adjustments for a minor chronic back complaint. I'd do a little gentle tweaking, and she'd be on her way, and I wouldn't see her again for another six months or so.

Margie wasn't in the office frequently enough for me to notice that she hadn't been in for a while. When I saw her name on my appointment list that day, I studied her chart and realized I hadn't seen her in over two years.

Because I'm trained to observe these things, when I walked into the examination room, I immediately detected that she was carrying an eighteen-month-old baby girl. Little Abby was an adorable bundle of energy with lots of smiles and baby giggles.

Not surprisingly, Margie's complaint was severe lower-back pain.

We discussed her working diagnosis based on her past medical history. I explained that it was very likely that the pregnancy and birth may have caused her existing back disorder to recur.

"She was born a year and a half ago," Margie reasoned. "I'm back to my weight before I was pregnant. It has to be something else."

I nodded, not conceding anything but sensing that I would be proven right. "First of all, can I ask you if there was a specific reason you stopped seeing me while you were pregnant?" I asked.

"Sure," she answered. "My obstetrician told me not to."

I did a double take and responded with a very doctorlike "Really?"

Margie went on to explain that when she complained of pelvic and lower-back pain during her pregnancy, her ob-gyn specifically instructed her not to come see me (her long-term chiropractor and a trained lower-back specialist).

At that point, I realized that she had simply been following "doctor's orders."

Margie was quick to explain that her obstetrician told her that, because her pregnancy had loosened her ligaments, chiropractic adjustments could possibly damage her joints.

I wish I could say I was stunned by this specific medical doctor's troubling lack of information and his shortage of data to support his position. As I will explain later in this book, there are many chiropractors who specialize in maternity care. We are trained to use appropriate, effective techniques that are very gentle to the pregnant body.

Margie's constant low-back pain during her pregnancy and after she gave birth made the case for me that I should have been on her health care team throughout.

As I took her medical history, I learned that she had a very long labor ending with an emergency caesarean section.

The day she came to see me, she was in a great deal of pain. She was also exhausted from getting up with feedings, and her lower back was "killing" her, further degrading her sleep.

Margie simply wasn't enjoying motherhood the way it was meant to be.

I examined her pelvis and lower back, and both were a mess (not a medical term)! Margie had multiple alignment problems of the pelvis and lower back. We knew that her back and pelvis were aligned the last time she was in my office. And we also knew that these pelvic misalignments were not caused by the birth itself because she eventually she had a C-section.

Could having massage, doing exercises and stretches, as well as receiving chiropractic care, acupuncture, and nutritional advice have helped her avoid having a C-section? I don't know because I was out of the loop for a couple of years. I can say that it is very probable that she would not have the type and severity of lower-back pain she was experiencing when she finally made it back into my office.

Margie is one of the reasons that I felt this book needed to be written: To empower women to choose how to treat their bodies during pregnancy based on good information. One of your fundamental rights as a patient is the right to decide what happens to your body. You need to gather all of the available information and make your own decision.

Margie is still a patient and has had another child with chiropractic care before and after giving birth. Her second baby was born vaginally.

What can you tell me about my back?

Your back is the focus of my training and my career. I can tell you more about your back than I'm sure you really want to know. Suffice it to say, your back is a critical component of your body, both structurally and functionally, in the role it plays by controlling all of the other parts that make up your physical being.

If you take your back out of commission, every other part of your body is negatively impacted.

If you break your arm, your body can compensate and keep doing what it's supposed to do. If you take your back out of commission, every other part of your body is negatively impacted.

Besides letting you stand erect, your spinal column encases your spinal cord, composed of central nervous system tissue that is essentially an extension of your brain. The nervous system either directly or indirectly controls or regulates all of the other systems in the body. Its impact is so far reaching that every hair on your body and every pore in your skin has a nerve going to it. A reaction as simple as goose bumps is controlled by nerves connected to your spinal cord.

The spinal cord is the body's information superhighway. In function, it serves as the brain's electrical conduit to the body's farthest extremities. The spinal cord itself consists of long nerve tracts encased in a hollow body chamber formed by the interlinked vertebrae of the spine. This delicate cordlike structure runs from your neck down to the beginning of your lower back. In vital brain-to-body communication, the spinal cord is the middleman. It relays messages between the brain and every organ of the body, including the heart, the blood vessels, the lungs, the kidneys, the intestines, and every one of the muscles in your body.

The back is not made up of a solid load-bearing bone. Much as a palm tree has to give in to the wind or snap, the spinal column also requires flexibility. The human body would never move freely—lean forward, arch backward, bend from side to side, or twist—if the back was rigid.

Much as a palm tree has to give in to the wind or snap, the spinal column also requires flexibility.

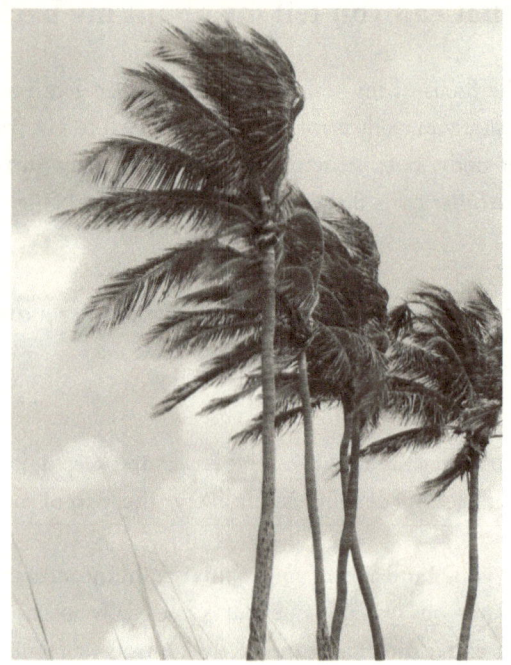

In order for body movement to occur, the back is comprised of a complex assembly incorporating multiple bones as well as discs, joints, ligaments, muscles, and nerves.

Part A of the appendix of this book gives you a brief but more in-depth lesson on *the anatomy of your back*.

Why can't I just take a painkiller for back pain?

Few doctors will prescribe any chemical intervention to relieve pain while you're pregnant. There's ample research available that suggests even something as seemingly mild as aspirin or acetaminophen (Tylenol) can adversely affect your baby.

Rather than prescribing a painkiller, some medical doctors choose to sidestep the question with the old line about a little back pain being part of pregnancy. Other more enlightened obstetricians might recommend an alternative form of care. And that's when moms-to-be get referred to chiropractors like me.

> **A note about pain:** Pain is your body's tool to let you know that something is wrong. Your body is warning you not to move in a certain way, for example, so that an injured part of your body is not further damaged and has a chance to heal. Painkillers block those messages. You get temporary relief from pain, but you risk causing greater damage because you have silenced the body's natural shout of caution.
>
> As an expectant mother, painkillers are rarely an option for mitigating back pain. That's why you need to avoid causing pain and, if that fails, find a way of alleviating the pain without swallowing a pill.

SECTION 2

BEFORE YOUR BABY'S BIRTHDAY

CHAPTER 3

YOUR HEALTH CARE TEAM

Whom can I consult to avoid or relieve back pain?

Although nothing is more natural than childbirth, nobody is born with all of the knowledge required to have a successful delivery. With most challenges in life, we learn by doing the old apprentice system. Success in sports is explained with three words: practice, practice, practice. With perhaps the most important event in your life, giving birth, you are remarkably ill prepared. And even if this isn't your first pregnancy, often, each prenatal and postnatal experience is different from child to child for the same mother.

You shouldn't try to tackle this event alone or with just your ob-gyn. Ideally, you should assemble a back-conscious health care team of pregnancy specialists. Your back may very well require the talents, skills, and ministrations of professionals from several disciplines. You should definitely start with your obstetrician, but if at all possible, you should add a chiropractor. As the need arises, he or she may refer you to a massage therapist, a physical therapist, an acupuncturist, or a nutritionist.

If they all end up on your team, it's an entourage worthy of a high-profile diva, but each highly trained specialist plays a vital role. And you deserve it.

You may not need the whole team for your entire pregnancy, but you need to be ready to call on them when the need arises. In many cases, your insurance will pay for some or all of the alternative-care options you need to avoid back pain.

For your back to be healthy and discomfort free, you need to put in some hard work and turn to experts for their expertise.

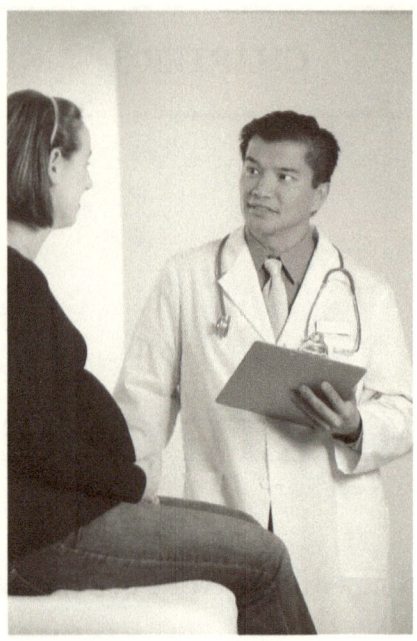

Why so many specialists, and what do they do?

The days of the GP, general practitioner, doctor who delivered babies, set broken bones, and took out your tonsils are long gone. Today we have cardiologists, podiatrists, neurologists, gastroenterologists, dermatologists, and basically more *ists* than you can shake a stick at. While it is reassuring to have a specialist for a specific medical need, we must realize that specializing in one area means that the other areas of the body are left to other specialists.

Your reproductive system isn't the only part of your body impacted by your pregnancy.

Your reproductive system isn't the only part of your body impacted by your pregnancy.

The team members I recommend are as follows:

Obstetrician

There's no argument that your ob-gyn medical doctor is the key member of your pregnancy health care team.

According to the Careers in Medicine Web site of the Association of American Medical Colleges: "An obstetrician/gynecologist possesses special knowledge, skills and professional capability in the medical and surgical care of the female reproductive system and associated disorders."

Note: There was no mention of your back and spinal column.

Just as you wouldn't go to a brain surgeon with a sore throat, when it comes to bringing your baby into the world, you want a doctor who graduated from medical school, served an internship, and then put in four years of residency and two additional clinical years of practice learning all that can be learned about bringing your baby out of your womb.

Your obstetrician has concentrated training specifically on your reproductive system.

Although every good ob-gyn physician will know something about back pain in pregnant patients because he/she has seen it during the course of treatment of other expectant mothers, your obstetrician has concentrated training specifically on your reproductive system. The doctor's waiting room is filled with women with the same wonderful condition that's happening between your ribs and your pelvis.

Your back is literally outside his/her specialty.

"Okay," you may ask, "why don't I just go to a back doctor?" A *back doctor* within the traditional medical community is a group of doctors called orthopedic surgeons. The last thing you want to do when you're pregnant is have a back operation. And honestly, rarely does back pain in pregnant women come from a surgically repairable condition.

The truth is treating back pain during pregnancy without medicine and without surgery is outside the expertise of medical doctors, leaving them to urge you to "tough it out." That's where the chiropractor becomes important.

Chiropractor

While medical doctors are primarily divided into two general categories, doctors who treat using medicine and doctors who treat using a scalpel, doctors of chiropractic use manipulation. We actually move parts around to put them back where they belong. A chiropractor manually adjusts the joints of the spine, allowing the nerves of the body to function properly.

The focus of our specialty is your back—your spinal column and the bones, joints, ligaments, muscles, and nerves that make up what we commonly think of as our back.

Chiropractic treatment involves manipulation and adjustment of the spinal column. The objective of a good chiropractor is to realign the body in a way that restores and preserves health without drugs or surgery. When you think it through, it makes sense that when your body is properly aligned the way it was designed, the various parts will work together more easily and without stress or pain.

The objective of a good chiropractor is to realign the body in a way that restores and preserves health without drugs or surgery.

No drugs.

No surgery.

A perfect combination for a pregnant woman with back pain.

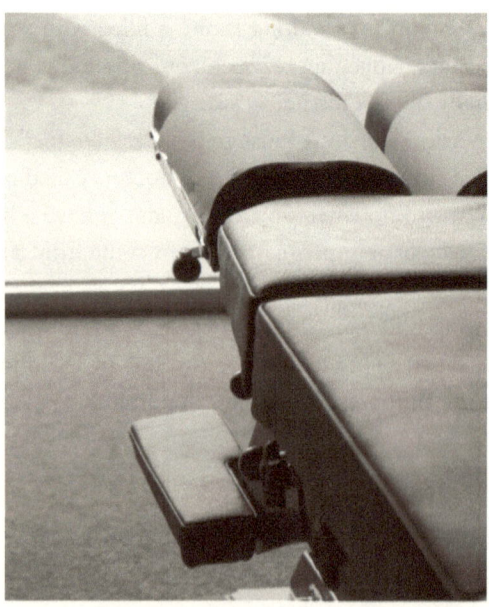

Aren't chiropractors quacks?

The quick answer is no, chiropractors are licensed doctors who have undergone rigorous schooling and adhere to strict professional standards.

For many years, though, there has been a degree of disdain within the traditional medical community toward doctors of chiropractic. In arrogant ignorance, some have called the profession *pseudoscience.*

In fact, to earn a doctor of chiropractic degree in most states, a student must have first earned a bachelor's degree just to get into a postgraduate program.

Students of chiropractic are required to take more hours of study in anatomy, physiology, and neurology than those in typical medical school programs.

Students of chiropractic are required to take more hours of study in anatomy, physiology, and neurology than those in typical medical school programs. During the first year of classroom training, a chiropractic student learns all about the basic sciences that are the foundation of chiropractic, such as anatomy, neurology, physiology, and chemistry along with pathology and bacteriology. In the second year of the curriculum, courses in diagnosis, chiropractic technique, and radiology are added. The third year is devoted to hands-on caring for patients in an outpatient clinic setting.

Nobody will dispute that there are chiropractors out there who should be looking for another line of work just as there are medical doctors who shouldn't be practicing medicine and lawyers who should be barred from the courtroom. Every profession has its share of underperformers.

You would be wise check out every member of your health care team. Just as it makes sense for you to have confidence in your ob-gyn, each of the other health care professionals you work with during your pregnancy should also inspire confidence. Often, one specialist you trust can refer you to someone in whom he or she has confidence. Other times, you may want to ask a friend or family member who has already gone through the experience.

Good or bad, every chiropractor will have a reputation in the community. Don't just search the local yellow pages, ask. Do your due diligence. I've encountered people who have searched harder for an auto mechanic than a health care professional. You deserve the best team you can assemble.

Another good rule of thumb is to pick a chiropractor who is a mother or a father—the more kids, the better. That way, you'll know that your chiropractor isn't just *book smart,* but actually has a wealth of firsthand experience dealing with precisely the issues that you're facing with your back pain.

What exactly will my chiropractor do for me?

That's a fair question. Your chiropractor will help keep your body aligned throughout your pregnancy.

During pregnancy, there are several physiological and endocrinological changes that occur inside you to get ready for delivering your developing baby. The changes can result in altering the alignment of your spine or the joints of your back. The conditions are as follows:

♦ protruding abdomen and increased back curve
♦ pelvic changes
♦ postural adaptations

Your body alignment, commonly referred to as your *posture*, is discussed in greater detail in chapter 6. But here's a quick overview: your body alignment is dependent on the *patency* of your spinal column. (*Patency* is a fancy medical term that means something is *open* or *unblocked*.) Your chiropractor aids in assuring spinal patency.

As your baby grows and your center of gravity changes, your chiropractor will adjust bones, joints, and ligaments to assure good posture and keep every affected part functioning as it's supposed to, pain free.

Chiropractic care will establish pelvic balance, which increases your baby's ability to move into the correct position for birth. In many cases, this avoids breech and posterior presentations and can eliminate the potential for *dystocia* (difficult labor). The end result is often an easier, safer delivery for both you and your baby.

Chiropractic care will establish pelvic balance, which increases your baby's ability to move into the correct position for birth.

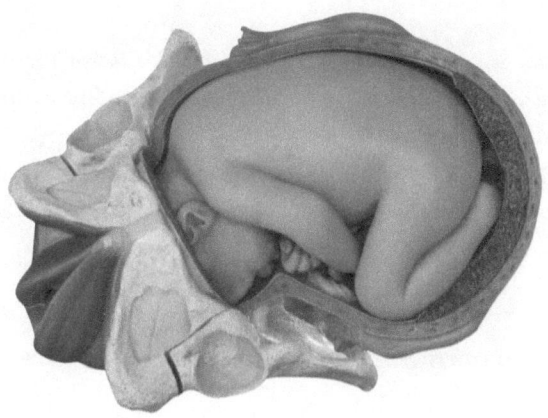

A chiropractor who is sensitive to a pregnant woman's needs will have special equipment for dealing with patients in your condition.

A good chiropractor will also advise you on everything from your pillow and sleeping position to the proper way to lift and carry your new baby's older sibling to minimize back strain and pain.

Your chiropractor will also recommend other health care professionals to work with during your pregnancy.

But is chiropractic care truly safe for me during pregnancy?

Often, after I've successfully helped relieve a pregnant woman of her back pain, she has confessed to being initially fearful that chiropractic would somehow be harmful to her baby.

You can stop worrying! A good chiropractor will help, not hurt. Okay, I'm a chiropractor, so I might be a little biased; so don't just take my word for it. According to the American Pregnancy Association (www.americanpregnancy.org), a national health organization committed to promoting reproductive and pregnancy wellness through education, research, advocacy, and community awareness: "There are NO contraindications to chiropractic care throughout pregnancy." (The capital letters are mine.)

(In *medicine*, a *contraindication* is a condition or factor that increases the *risks* involved in using a particular *drug*, carrying out a medical procedure, or engaging in a particular activity.)

So according to the American Pregnancy Association, there is no reason *not* to seek chiropractic care anytime during pregnancy. And notice, they used the word *throughout* pregnancy.

There are no contraindications to chiropractic care throughout pregnancy.

—American Pregnancy Association

It should be noted that the medical advisory board of the association includes eighteen medical doctors, many of whom teach reproductive medicine at some of the nation's leading medical schools. *There are no chiropractors on the advisory board.*

The American Pregnancy Association lists the following potential benefits of chiropractic care during pregnancy:

- maintaining a healthier pregnancy
- controlling symptoms of nausea
- increasing the likelihood of full-term delivery
- reducing the time of labor and delivery
- relieving back, neck, or joint pain
- preventing a potential caesarean section

Despite such a glowing endorsement, for some reason not supported by empirical or clinical data, many traditional doctors have the misconception that a chiropractor "cracks" your bones and "twists" your body into awkward and damaging positions. I once heard an actor portraying a medical doctor on television refer to chiropractic care as "unwarranted trauma to the body."

Ouch. That statement was not only wrong, but shamefully uninformed.

I wouldn't let anyone, no matter what degrees were hanging on his or her wall, *crack* or *twist* my wife's body, whether she was pregnant or not. My wife, Gina, had chiropractic care with all four of our kids.

In the real world, a chiropractor doesn't manipulate or force your body to do anything it wasn't designed to do. I'll bet that any medical doctor who has negative comments about doctors of chiropractic can't even name four of the nearly one hundred chiropractic techniques, let alone explain how pelvic balance is imperative for an easy labor.

In the real world, the chiropractor doesn't manipulate or force your body to do anything it wasn't designed to do.

A fact that I always find edifying is that chiropractors as a group pay significantly less for malpractice insurance than other health care professionals, especially medical doctors. Everyone who has ever bought insurance knows that greater risks require higher insurance premiums. If a chiropractor was more dangerous than a medical doctor, wouldn't we be paying more for malpractice insurance than your ob-gyn does? Ask a skeptical medical doctor to explain why just the opposite is true.

BREATHLESS REFERRAL

It was in the heat of the summer when a mother-to-be was referred to our office by her obstetrician. Cindy was in her thirty-sixth week, about four weeks prior to delivery. It seems Cindy had gone for her checkup with her ob-gyn and complained of a sharp, shooting pain from her midback to her sternum (breastbone) on the right side of her body.

"I can't breathe," she explained somewhat breathlessly.

The first thing to consider with that kind of complaint is the gallbladder. Her ob-gyn gave her a thorough examination and eliminated her gallbladder as the culprit. The doctor could find no other cause for the pain.

Fortunately, for Cindy, her ob-gyn resisted the typical MD diagnosis of a "muscle strain" and, instead, recommended that she see a chiropractor, specifically me.

I quickly ascertained that not only hadn't Cindy ever seen a chiropractor before, she didn't have a clue as to what I could possibly do to help her. I had my work cut out for me just establishing my credibility.

Cindy is a petite woman, and she was carrying a large baby. The medical term we use in my office is **all belly.**

In taking her history, I learned that Cindy had not been experiencing significant lower-back or pelvic pain throughout her pregnancy. Of course, she did point out that her feet hurt and her back "got tired," but what pregnant woman doesn't have the same complaint?

The recent pain that affected her breathing came on suddenly. As she described it, "It feels like someone is putting an ice pick in my back." Ouch.

She explained that the pain had started about a week and a half earlier, and she remembered first noticing it when she rolled over in bed. Initially, the discomfort was a jabbing pain right of center in her midback. It had progressed to wrapping around her sternum, primarily on the right side.

Hmmm.

I examined her and discovered what I had expected to find after her description. Cindy was suffering from a costovertebral subluxation.

"A what?" she asked.

I explained that, in layman's terms, she had a rib out of place. I surmised that what had happened was that a combination of the increased size of the baby in the late third trimester, the labored breathing that accompanies the large baby pressing against her internal organs, and the natural loosening of the ligaments caused by the hormones released during pregnancy made it possible to knock the rib slightly out of place when she rolled over in bed.

The explanation made sense to Cindy, and she nodded her head in understanding. "So now what?" she asked.

After a few minutes of gentle adjustments working on her rib cage and midback, she felt instant relief.

You've gotta love it when that happens.

This was a great example of an obstetrician working with a chiropractor for the good of the patient and her baby. Instead of Cindy enduring considerable discomfort through the last month of her pregnancy with severe rib pain and gasping for breath, I put in a couple of minutes on the table, and she enjoyed relief.

From knowing nothing about chiropractors and even being a little hesitant about her visit to my office, Cindy has become one of my best referral sources. She sends people to me all of the time.

Physical therapist

Let's say for a moment that you're told that you're going to have to carry around a thirty-pound weight for 280 days, 24/7 with no relief. And you can't use your hands!

After finishing a period of denial that may or may not include some unattractive whining, your first thought will be a panicked "I've gotta get in shape!" That's actually a great idea. Unfortunately, by the time you find out you're going to need to get ready for this ordeal, it has already started; and there's no turning back.

By the time you find out you're going to need to get ready for this ordeal, it has already started, and there's no turning back.

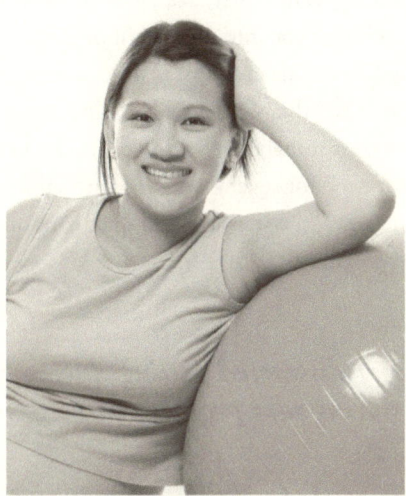

That's where a physical therapist or personal athletic trainer comes in. Just as it makes perfect sense to get your body ready, it's great to know that exercising has also been found to be a great natural remedy for back pain.

Physical therapy (or physiotherapy) is the health care specialty that helps people develop, maintain, and restore maximum movement and functional ability. Your physical therapist is concerned with identifying and maximizing movement potential. As a pregnant woman, your goal is to improve musculature without a rigorous exercise regimen because that may do more harm than good.

Is physical therapy safe for me during pregnancy?

Obviously, there are activities that you should refrain from doing while you're pregnant. Anything involving contact, stress, twisting, the potential for falling, or extreme exertion should be avoided. But unless you have extenuating medical circumstances, exercise will usually help prevent back pain by strengthening the muscles that support the back. An added advantage is that exercise can help improve circulation, which helps prevent leg cramps, swelling of the ankles, constipation, hemorrhoids, and varicose veins.

Of course, you should check with your doctor before starting an exercise program, even under the careful eye of a trained physical therapist or personal athletic trainer. For most women, exercise is very beneficial. But for women who have a high-risk pregnancy or are at risk for preterm labor, exercise should be closely monitored.

Massage therapist

Be ready for the argument, "But, honey, I can give you a back rub." Remember, that's being said by the same guy who got you into this condition in the first place. Fifteen minutes of distracted petting during *SportsCenter* a couple of times during your pregnancy isn't gonna to cut it. Explain to the poor guy that what he'd be doing would be like playing catch in the backyard. What you need is somebody playing shortstop in Yankee Stadium.

You need an hour at a time for several sessions throughout your pregnancy with a trained specialist. In many cases, the massage therapist is second in importance only to your ob-gyn during your pregnancy.

Fifteen minutes of distracted petting during **SportsCenter** *a couple of times during your pregnancy isn't gonna to cut it.*

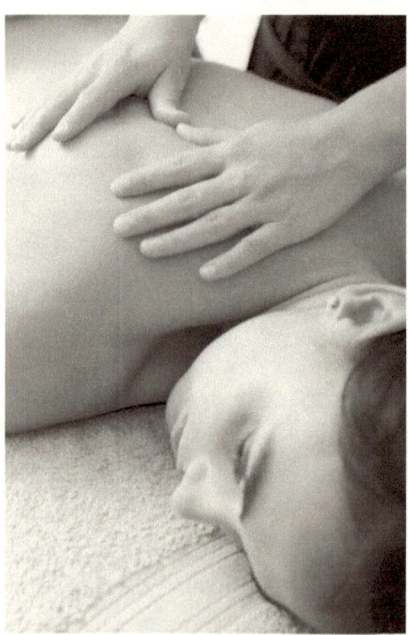

Choose a massage therapist who has a minimum of fifteen hundred class hours or a special degree specifically in pregnancy massage. A massage therapist who specializes in pregnant women will have special equipment to accommodate your condition. This will include a table with the stomach area cut out or a Prego Pillow, a large donut-shaped pillow that you can put your stomach in.

Your ob-gyn or your chiropractor should know the top pregnancy massage therapists in your area. Expect someone with an office that obviously caters to pregnant women. As a general rule, the better the massage therapist, the harder it will be to get an appointment.

Today's expectant mothers are frequently working full-time, and many already have children making demands on their time and body. Exhaustion is common. Having a professional massage is a wonderful and passive way to keep all of your tendons, ligaments, and muscles stretched and moving. These healing hands go a long way in preventing many of the pitfalls that cause mechanical lower-back problems.

Here are some benefits of prenatal massage:

- neck and back pain relief caused by muscle imbalance and weakness
- assistance in maintaining proper posture
- lessened sciatic pain
- stress relief on weight-bearing joints, such as lower back, pelvis, and ankles
- preparation of the muscles used during childbirth
- fewer cramps
- emotional support and nurturing touch
- relaxation and decreased insomnia
- headache and sinus-congestion relief

Most women also appreciate the connection a massage makes between their body and their baby, not to mention the fact that it just makes you feel good. I've seen many women who feel sexier and happier with their beautiful pregnant bodies after a good massage. Dads will never understand the importance of this experience, but they can usually appreciate the results.

Eight massages before giving birth and another eight after the birth should make a major impact on your back health.

"Eight massages?" you may ask. "How am I going to afford eight massages? They aren't covered by my insurance."

You're right, of course. Insurance companies aren't overly concerned with your pain, so massage therapy may very well come out of pocket. But let's see for a moment whether you can afford a massage a month. If a typical therapeutic massage is, say, sixty dollars an hour, you're looking at putting aside two dollars a day. Since your ob-gyn probably has you off coffee, that means the money you'll save by staying away from Starbucks will amount to about two dollars a day. There you go! You've paid for your massages without impacting the family budget.

But is massage therapy safe for me during pregnancy?

Massage administered by a therapist trained to care for pregnant women can be extremely safe. Again, you should check with your ob-gyn before starting massage treatments, but enlightened medical doctors are generally quite supportive of the concept.

There are some conditions to watch for that *may* exclude an expectant mother from massage. They include the following:

♦   heavy discharge (watery or bloody)
♦   diabetes
♦   any malignant condition
♦   contagious illness
♦   fever
♦   vomiting
♦   abdominal pain
♦   preeclampsia high blood
♦   pressure
♦   diarrhea
♦   morning sickness
♦   unusual pain

In my practice, I rarely recommend massage therapy during the first trimester simply because your body generally doesn't need any extra stimulation at that time.

Acupuncturist

"Why would I have anything to do with Chinese medicine featuring the word *puncture* during my pregnancy?" you may ask.

I've become convinced over the past several years that an acupuncturist can make a significant positive impact on your pregnancy throughout all nine months but especially during the third trimester.

As reported in the journal *Birth*, acupuncture can help alleviate things like morning sickness and severe bouts of vomiting known as *hyperemesis gravidarum*.

Acupuncture can help alleviate things like morning sickness and severe bouts of vomiting.

I have also seen acupuncture therapy successfully treat loss of energy, insomnia, and night sweats. (It is also frequently used to help relieve hemorrhoids, heartburn, and edema.)

The focus of this book is your back, of course; and experience has shown that acupuncture has frequently proven valuable in treating *sciatica*, which is pain that radiates from your back through your buttocks, thigh, leg, and even your foot in some cases.

Your acupuncturist will insert hair-thin needles under your skin. The needles usually stay in for fifteen to twenty minutes. Little or no discomfort is experienced from having the needles inserted. Pain relief is suspected to come from the release of endorphins, the human body's natural painkillers.

Back in 1998, the National Institutes of Health concluded that acupuncture might help conditions that involve chronic back pain, including low-back pain.

What's one good reason for me to let someone stick me with a pin?

When you're a week past your due date and maybe a little cranky, this piece of advice may well be worth the price of this book.

Since nothing does more for relieving back pain from pregnancy than the actual childbirth, acupuncture is of special interest after your pregnancy has gone into overtime. Throughout my career, I've had expectant moms come to me and report that all is well with the baby, but the little rascal is a little reluctant to make his or her debut.

That's when I often recommend the acupuncturist.

I've seen many cases over the years when an acupuncturist was actually able to "speed up the baby." In fact, you can often avoid chemically inducing labor because your acupuncturist has the knowledge and ability to stimulate normal contractions and "kick-start" your body to begin the birthing process.

The most significant clinical treatment I have witnessed firsthand, though, has been acupuncture's success in turning breech babies. I have had chiropractic success using Webster technique among others, but I will usually step aside if an acupuncturist is available. What a good acupuncturist can do is nothing short of amazing. I have found it to consistently be simple, safe, and effective.

Of course, with a breech situation, I work closely with the ob-gyn to make sure the placenta or cord is not impeding the baby's position before turning the baby either chiropractically or in concert with an acupuncturist.

Your chiropractor can usually refer you to a good acupuncturist.

THE BREECH BABY AND THE MUGWORT

I know, the title of this anecdote sounds like the next installment in the Harry Potter series. Technically, it really isn't a back story, but it should give you a good idea about how the various members of your back health care team can work together for you and your baby during your pregnancy.

A local midwife referred a woman carrying a breech baby to our office. I'll call the expectant mom Jennifer. She was in her thirty-seventh week, and there was no mistaking the fact that the baby's head was pointing 180 degrees in the wrong direction.

Jennifer was conflicted. She had never seen a chiropractor before and didn't seem overly enthusiastic about being in my office. The other side of her dilemma was that she clearly wanted to avoid a caesarean section if at all possible. It was obvious to me that she would do anything within reason for her baby. So there we were.

The referring midwife was aware that I had become something of an authority on turning breech babies. As a side story to this side story, my second child, Olivia, was in a breech position as late as the fortieth week. I was a very young chiropractor and knew the theory about turning babies, but I didn't have the clinical experience I needed to do the job right. I enlisted the aid of the chiropractor's version of Yoda (note the Star Wars *reference), an older talented, more experienced doctor whom I respected. I did a crash apprenticeship under the guidance of the old pro, and Olivia flipped in about thirty-six hours, plenty of time for a normal birth experience for mother and daughter.*

Since that blessed event, I have gained a tremendous amount of clinical experience with pregnant moms facing a possible breech birth. Soon, I'll be looked at as the crotchety old mentor with all of the knowledge.

Now back to Jennifer's story. I worked up her medical history and learned that she had some minor lower-back pain during this, her second pregnancy. She had a slight pelvic misalignment that I was able to correct with a gentle adjustment. Jennifer was physically fit, and a check of her ultrasound revealed that the umbilical cord was not wrapped around the baby's neck.

After I had all of the diagnostic ammunition I needed, I did something that many readers might find surprising: I recommended she see our acupuncturist.

I realized that Jennifer didn't come into my office very confident that I could help her resolve her breech situation. Frankly, I sensed I was her last resort. And now I was recommending that she go to an even less traditional health care practitioner.

Why? you may ask. Because it was the right thing to do in her case.

Looking back at it now, I can appreciate that Jennifer was a very brave woman. In her position, I don't know that I could have managed her courage.

Remarkably, she didn't run screaming from my office when I told her I wanted her to visit the acupuncturist so he could burn a mugwort herb (Artemisia vulgaris) *on her pinky toe. "Mugwort?" you may be wondering. "Are you nuts?" C'mon. It's no weirder than a pedicure.*

The procedure doesn't use needles and is referred to as moxibustion. You may never have heard of it, but there's speculation in the Chinese medical community that moxibustion was first used shortly after humans became aware of fire. What do you call something that's a whole lot older than ancient?

I was a little apprehensive about Jennifer's reaction to burning mugwort therapy, but she took it like a trooper. In fact, she admitted to having read about it that very morning when she did an Internet search for flipping a breech baby.

I nearly dislocated my jaw when my mouth dropped in surprise.

I assured her that the smoldering herb would never be closer than an inch from her skin. It burns above the skin, causing no damage or injury. She said, "Let's do it," and marched in to meet the acupuncturist.

He did moxibustion over her pinky toe in brief sessions over two days, and the baby turned.

Jennifer had a wonderful delivery. And I have a great story to tell about a woman who was nervous about so-called alternative medicine but loved her baby so much that she was willing to try something that sounds pretty bizarre to most of us.

But is acupuncture safe for me and my baby?

Acupuncture has been used for treating nausea and low-back pain among other ailments in China since at least the Han dynasty (206 BC to AD 220), and there is evidence that a form of the treatment was used as many as fifty-two hundred years ago. Naturally, you would have to assume that anything that has been practiced for thousands of years has to have a fairly good track record.

Recently, many health insurance companies have begun recognizing acupuncture as a legitimate treatment not only for pain relief, but also as a treatment for nausea in early pregnancy.

About ten years ago, the American Medical Association called for stringently controlled research of acupuncture and other so-called alternative therapies. Your baby may be a doctor himself before the AMA makes a definitive ruling concerning acupuncture. However, a European survey by Ernst et al. published in 2003 studied over four hundred patients receiving over thirty-five hundred acupuncture treatments. The research found that the most common adverse effects of acupuncture were as follows:

- ◆ minor bleeding after removal of the needles, roughly 3 percent of patients
- ◆ hematoma (minor bruising), about 2 percent of patients
- ◆ dizziness (usually attributed to anxiety), about 1 percent of patients

Two combined studies in the United Kingdom covering 66,229 acupuncture treatments yielded only 134 minor adverse events (*British Medical Journal*, 2001 September 1). There were no major adverse effects reported.

In hospitals in the United States in 1994, there were 2.216 million *serious* adverse drug reactions according to a 1998 article in the *Journal of the American Medical Association*.

So statistically, you have a 0.02 percent chance of having a minor adverse effect with acupuncture. Using prescription medications in a hospital environment, you have a 6.7 percent chance of experiencing a serious adverse event.

Statistically, you have a 0.02 percent chance of having a minor adverse effect with acupuncture. Using prescription medications in a hospital environment, you have a 6.7 percent chance of experiencing a serious adverse event.

Nutritionist

A bad diet during pregnancy often leads to lower-back pain. A nutritionist is a great resource for dietary modification during pregnancy, impacting both the mom and the baby. Expect the nutritionist to increase protein and restrict fat, sodium, caffeine, and preservatives, which lead to swelling, water retention, and lethargy.

Lethargy leads to skipping exercises, which leads to weight gain, which invariably leads to lower-back pain.

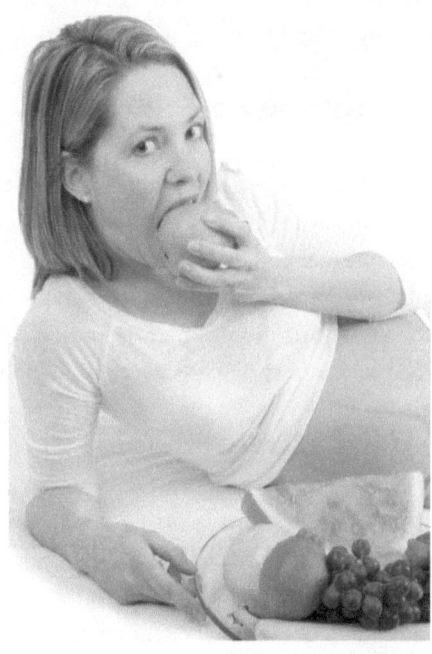

Bad diets can also cause gallbladder inflammation and its resultant midback pain. Headaches are also very common with dehydration.

Many ob-gyn practices have a dietician on staff. If not, either your ob-gyn or one of the other members of your health care team can refer you to a good prenatal nutritionist.

Are all of these therapies safe for me and my baby?

Nothing I've suggested has proven to have a negative impact on either the mother or the baby—no contraindications. It's not an unusual question, though. Toning your muscles (physical therapist) and eating the right foods (nutritionist) just makes good sense. The question is most frequently asked about the other specialties. Hopefully, I've been able to debunk some myths and give you some insight.

Can a midwife be a member of my team?

Absolutely. It's your choice. Many of my pregnant patients come to me through the recommendations of a midwife. Because midwives are concerned with things like nutrition and exercise, pregnancy health, breast-feeding, and quality infant care, noninvasive specialties like chiropractic care, massage therapy, and acupuncture are all in keeping with the midwives' efforts to minimize technological interventions.

Of my four children, one was born under the care of a midwife.

What exactly is a midwife?

A midwife is a health care professional who provides an array of health-oriented services for women that may include medical histories, gynecological examinations, and labor and delivery care.

Specific services of a modern-day midwife depend on the individual's certification and licensure credentials and the practice restrictions within each state in the United States.

From ancient times up to the eighteenth century in Western culture, the care of mothers and delivery of infants was regarded, both by patients and by the medical profession, as appropriately carried out by women referred to as *midwives*.

References to midwives are found in ancient Hindu records, in Greek and Roman manuscripts, and even in the Bible.

> *And as she was having great difficulty in childbirth, the midwife said to her, "Don't be afraid, for you have another son."*
>
> —Genesis 35:17

> *So God was kind to the midwives and the people increased and became even more numerous. And because the midwives feared God, he gave them families of their own.*
>
> —Exodus 1:20-21

It wasn't until the middle of the eighteenth century that childbirth became primarily the providence of medical doctors. The first school of midwifery in the United States opened in 1933. Today in Europe, midwives participate in approximately 70 percent of all births. In the United States, that figure is closer to 10 percent.

The major difference between doctors and midwives is that doctors are taught to *manage* pregnancy and childbirth while midwives *assist*. Doctors are also able to intervene surgically when necessary as well as administer drugs and anesthetics.

When is using a midwife appropriate?

Midwives are an option with low-risk pregnancies, which make up 60 to 80 percent of all pregnancies. The downside is if you fall in that 20 to 40 percent of pregnancies where either the mother or the baby will require medical intervention that is outside the services offered by a midwife. Unfortunately, it's not always clear in which group you belong.

If complications are anticipated, I recommend you choose a hospital setting where there is ready access to obstetricians, perinatologists, pediatricians, and other experts as well as all of the whistles and bells needed to deal with a variety of difficulties.

Throughout the remainder of this book, whenever I refer to your ob-gyn, *feel free to substitute* midwife *if that is the decision you've made.*

CHAPTER 4

YOUR BACK PAIN (PART 1)

What causes back pain specific to pregnant women?

There are two areas that can cause back pain in pregnant women: pathological and musculoskeletal.

Pathological causes of back pain include back ailments that have occurred or would have occurred independent of the pregnancy, like herniated discs. They also include disease processes of the organs such as kidney stones, endometriosis, fibroid tumors, ectopic pregnancy, and implantation of the embryo in the uterine wall.

The majority of pregnant women, though, suffer back pain because of the body mechanics involved in compensating for the weight of the baby and the shift in the mother's center of gravity. These musculoskeletal causes are a result of your body's physical inability to offset the dynamic growing miracle balanced above your pelvis. The result is that you end up with a sore back.

Musculoskeletal back pain is the focus of this book.

Because carrying the baby will alter both your posture and your movement, even a professional dancer or a world-class gymnast is challenged to be graceful while pregnant.

What are the most common kinds of musculoskeletal back pain during pregnancy?

Most doctors agree that there are three common types of back pain during pregnancy:

1. lumbar pain—in the lumbar vertebrae in your lower back
2. posterior and anterior pelvic pain—in the back and front of your pelvis
3. upper-back pain—in the thoracic spine area located above your lumbar area, just above where your ribs start

Lumbar pain is similar to the low-back pain you may have experienced before you were pregnant. You'll feel it over and around your spine, approximately at the level of your waist. You may also have pain that radiates to your buttocks, thighs, legs, feet, and pelvis that originates in the lumbar spine as nerve root irritation. Sitting or standing for long periods of time and lifting usually make this pain worse, and it tends to be more intense at the end of the day.

Posterior and anterior pelvic pain is most prevalent in the second and third trimester due to stretching ligaments. It is more an annoying, distracting ache that comes and goes rather than an intense pain. You may experience it at the top of your buttocks, above the bumps on your backside, or in the front, over the round ligaments to the center of the pubic bone.

Pelvic pain may be triggered by activities like walking, climbing stairs, getting in and out of the bathtub or a low chair, rolling over in bed, twisting, or lifting—basically anything physical you ordinarily do in the course of your day-to-day activities.

Most often, you feel pelvic pain bilaterally, or on both sides. The skeletal structures involved are at the level of the ilium or the sacrum.

Because the pelvis is the skeletal structure of the birthing canal, it has been my clinical experience that a woman with untreated pelvic pain is more likely to have trouble with the birthing process.

Because the pelvis is the skeletal structure of the birthing canal, . . . a woman with untreated pelvic pain is more likely to have trouble with the birthing process.

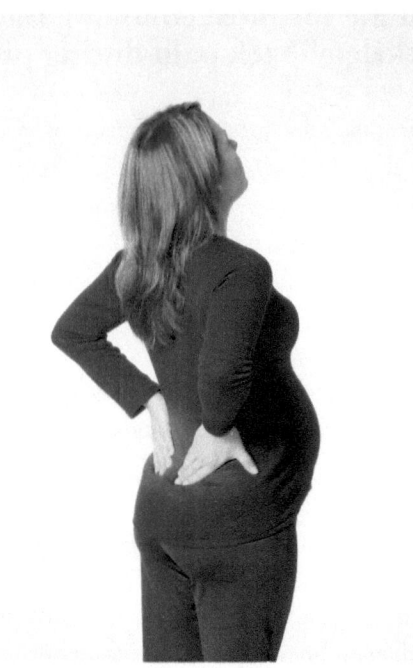

Upper-back pain is technically considered thoracic spine pain. This pain is most often felt around the area of your bra strap when you're pregnant. Many factors can contribute to this pain, some of which could be associated with the trauma that comes with morning sickness.

Pain in your upper back can be made worse as your ribs spread in the second and third trimesters as your baby grows. Typically, during this time in your pregnancy, your respiration is also affected as well as your rib angles.

Change in your breast size can also contribute to upper-back pain.

Although upper-back pain is the least common type of musculoskeletal back pain associated with pregnancy, it can be one of the most intense. The good news is that upper-back pain is typically the easiest to resolve with chiropractic and massage treatments.

One caution, though, is that your diagnostician needs to differentiate upper-back pain from pain caused by your gallbladder.

HEARTBURN HOTEL

Back pain isn't the only result of your organs being smushed up by your growing baby. There's also heartburn. Not genteel, well-mannered heartburn. We're talking about the kind of acid indigestion that can melt metal.

Marcia was a patient who had a doozy of a case of heartburn while she was pregnant. It was later in her pregnancy, where her organs were smashed up into her chest.

I had been taking care of Marcia throughout her pregnancy and dealt with some minor aches and pains through her first two trimesters. During the third trimester, she really started to show. She was in great shape, but there was a whole lot of baby entering a room long before the rest of her got there.

Marcia was committed to continuing her walking and stretching regardless of how big she got, but she kept getting terrible heartburn. She reported heartburn even when she wasn't eating. In addition to the stomach indigestion, Marcia was also suffering a "supertight" midback.

During one of our scheduled appointments, I concentrated on her midback and found several tight areas and misaligned joints. Although you'll probably never hear this diagnosis from a medical doctor, I explained to Marcia how the nerves of the stomach come from the sympathetic nervous system (spine) off the midback (specifically T5-7).

I went on to explain that due to the pressure the baby was putting on the stomach, stomach acid was being forced into her esophagus, causing her heartburn.

The heartburn, in turn, excites nerves to the spinal cord, causing muscle tightness in her midback due to the reflexive actions of the autonomic nervous system.

I showed Marcia a Meric chart of the spinal nerves. Then I did a very simple traction adjustment to her thoracic spine.

Marcia noted that the correction felt great. I asked her to come back in couple days for a recheck.

When she arrived, Marcia reported that her heartburn was "almost gone" and that I was "her hero."

Marcia was able to manage her heartburn with just a couple flare-ups through the end of her pregnancy and did very well with a few minor spinal corrections. Her medical doctor pooh-poohed my diagnosis and treatment, but Marcia was pleased and appreciative that we were able to eliminate her heartburn.

VISCERAL ISSUES VERSUS MECHANICAL ISSUES

Chiropractic care is not always the answer when you come into my office uttering the words, "My back is killing me." That statement is usually followed with a question like, "Is there anything you can do?"

This is a very familiar phrase with pregnant women, especially in their third trimester. And the truth is I can usually help . . . but not always.

Take the case of Lisa. Lisa had been a long-term patient, pregnant in her second trimester when she came into the office complaining of a stubborn and diffuse lower-back pain. I had been treating Lisa throughout her pregnancy and long before she and her husband, Todd, decided to start a family; so I was somewhat surprised that she developed such a pronounced back ailment without any warning signs.

I immediately did a thorough exam, and she showed very few and very minor alignment issues. I referred her to our massage therapist for a couple of massages and scheduled her for a return appointment three days later.

Lisa had her massages and reported that she felt much better. Two days after we thought we had conquered the problem, she was back in the office for an unscheduled appointment with me. Again, she was experiencing very uncomfortable pain over her lower back.

If she hadn't been pregnant, I would have sent Lisa for x-rays of her spine. I reexamined her, looking for something that I may have missed and did some further orthopedic testing. That was when she reported two things that she didn't believe were connected to her back pain: (1) she had a slight fever, and (2) there was tenderness over her flank area.

My diagnosis changed immediately. I was convinced that she had kidney stones. That meant an emergency visit to her obstetrician for an ultrasound.

She came back to me as soon as the diagnosis was confirmed. She indeed had kidney stones.

Lisa explained that her obstetrician had given some heavy-duty painkillers for when things got bad. Reluctant to put a prescription drug in her system, Lisa asked me what I could do.

I explained that kidney stones weren't something I could resolve chiropractically. "I can pray they go away," I offered.

Lisa just shook her head and smiled courageously. "Doctor, you are just no help at all."

What is sciatica?

There's a *buzzword* for you: a great many patients come into my office complaining of *sciatica*. In my clinical experience, *sciatica* is more often a general, imprecise term used to describe any pain along the buttock, posterior thigh, and leg. Much like *bellyache* or *headache*, *sciatica* is often used to describe where pain is occurring rather that what's actually causing it.

In my experience, true sciatica occurs when the piriformis muscle, which lies deep below the gluteal muscles, irritates the sciatic nerve, which emerges from the bottom of your pelviws. The medical term for this condition is *piriformis syndrome*, and the referred pain is correctly called *sciatica*. (You can read a more detailed explanation in appendix C in the back of this book.)

With true sciatica, patients generally complain of pain deep in the buttocks, which is made worse by activities like sitting and climbing stairs. The pain often goes down the back of the thigh or into the lower back.

Piriformis syndrome of the sciatic nerve is common during your last trimester because the deep ligaments of the pelvis loosen and stretch as the pelvis changes shape. This, in turn, also stretches the piriformis muscle, causing a pinching motion over the sciatic nerve.

Often, pain described as sciatica is actually nerve root entrapment at the spine caused by spinal pathologies like disc herniation or *foraminal stenosis*, both of which also can occur during pregnancy. Another condition frequently referred to as sciatica occurs when your baby compress the lumbosacral plexus in your last trimester. (The lumbosacral plexus is the group of nerve roots that combine like a river's tributaries to form the sciatic nerve.)

The bottom line is that your ob-gyn usually doesn't have the tools in his or her toolbox to deal with sciatic pain. They can urge you to "deal with it" as part of your pregnancy. But this is precisely where the body mechanics—your chiropractor, massage therapist, physical therapist, and acupuncturist—working on your health care team can help. Your alternative medicine team members have the training and expertise to figure out the cause of your pain and, in most cases, deal with it for you.

Even a stubborn baby sitting on your nerves in your pelvis can be moved to take the pressure off and relieve your pain.

What does it mean when my baby is "sitting on the nerves" in my pelvis?

It's a fairly common complaint I hear several times a week: "I've got pain over my buttocks and the front of my thighs. My doctor told me the baby is 'sitting on the nerves' in my pelvis."

What your ob-gyn is referring to is pressure on the *lumbosacral plexus*. The lumbosacral plexus is formed where the nerves branch off your lumbar spine and form a bundle or group of nerves in the interior of your pelvis.

What happens, especially in your third trimester, is your baby lies on the interior of your pelvis; and you experience pain over your lower back, anterior thigh, abdomen, and buttocks. This pain is usually diffuse (widespread) and intermittent (comes and goes with positioning).

There's not much your ob-gyn can do about the condition, but other members of your health care team can help move the baby off of the lumbosacral plexus. A visit to your chiropractor is a good starting place.

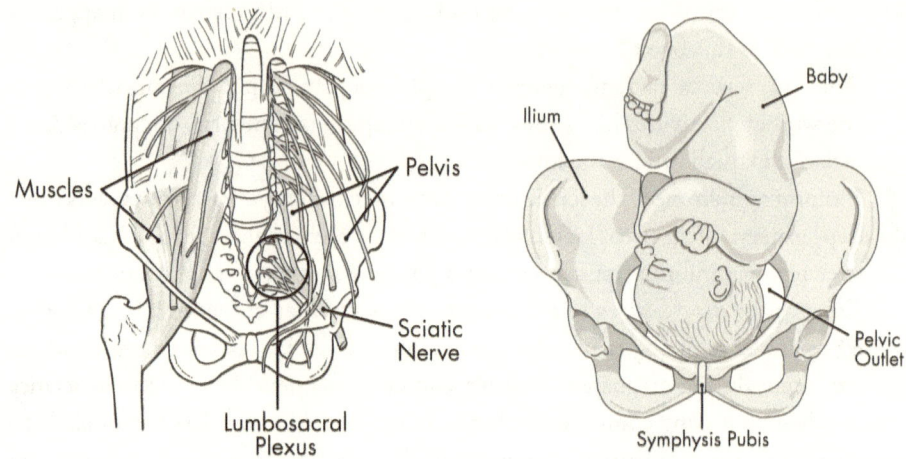

SCIATICA BY ANY OTHER NAME IS STILL A PAIN IN THE BUTT

A new patient came to see me just as I was writing this chapter. We'll call her Jill. As I'm writing this, she is thirty-three years old and fifteen weeks' pregnant. Jill was accompanied by two lovely young ladies. The older girl, Melanie, is almost four; and her sister, Bobbi, is just about to turn two years old.

Jill brought her stroller in instead of the car seat for Bobbi, the mark of a seasoned mom. Jill was also clearly in pain as she walked into the examination room.

As Jill started to fill me in on her condition, I learned that she had was experiencing moderate lower-back pain, but she was also dealing with a shooting sharp pain that burned into her left "hip" (the ilium-buttock area for those of you keeping score at home). The pain radiated down the back and side of her thigh.

Jill shared with me that she suffered lower-back pain with both Melanie and Bobbi but never had pain that shot into her thigh.

I explained that it is not uncommon after multiple births to have progressively worse lower-back pain, especially if untreated, ignored, or misdiagnosed. Why? Because of all the lifting, carrying, bending, bathing, cleaning, and diaper-changing activity that she had been doing with the other children over the past four years long before she became pregnant with the baby she was carrying.

I wished, not for the first time, that I had a copy of the book finished so I could give it to her. I think it was the sixteenth-century English philosopher Francis Bacon who first observed "Knowledge is power."

Jill's health history revealed that she was like many mothers today. She was unable to engage in any kind of exercise regimen due to a grueling work schedule and to her maternal and spousal duties.

I examined her thoroughly and, after orthopedic and neurological testing, determined that she suffered from nerve root irritation with probable disc involvement.

Jill didn't immediately accept the diagnosis, asking, "Nerves? Why does my butt muscle hurt? It must be more muscular."

I explained that when the nerves of the spine are irritated, they send a message to the brain. The brain, in turn, tells the muscles to splint the affected or dysfunctional area. We know this is happening when muscles in the affected area tighten. Nine times out of ten, this condition is misdiagnosed as some sort of muscle strain.

What actually happens is, on orders from the brain, a nerve-produced muscle spasm occurs to protect a nerve. It has nothing to do with a direct muscular injury. But because the muscles have been contracted in a spasm on only one side, she experienced pelvic misalignment and muscle pain.

While Jill's mind was processing this information, I referred her straight to the acupuncturist in our office. I chose acupuncture from my care "toolbox" because we needed to reset and calm down the nerve-produced muscle spasm in her thigh and buttocks.

Massage is often an alternative, but since I deemed Jill's case severe, I determined that acupuncture would require less force and still be very effective.

After four sessions of acupuncture, Jill's pain level and muscle spasms dropped to a 1 on a scale of 1 to 10.

I corrected the alignment issue of her pelvis, and Jill is finally enjoying motherhood again.

Because of Jill's work schedule, she couldn't maintain her level of improvement on her own. Her health care team needed to do their jobs, and she needed to participate in the process, not do all of the work on her own.

Jill is keeping regular appointments and still writing questions for me to answer. I love it.

What's your opinion on a sacroiliac belt?

At some point, your ob-gyn might suggest what's called a *sacroiliac belt* or an *SI joint belt*. This is an external belt that holds up your baby-filled stomach to take pressure off your sacroiliac joint, sort of like a support bra for your pelvis.

I've seen studies reporting the pros of using these devices as well as studies stating the cons.

I can see where using these belts for part of the day—when you're working at a physically demanding activity, for example—might have merit in relieving stress on your back. But I have to caution you that anytime you obstruct the natural function with an external apparatus, you run the risk of interfering with your body's physical processes. With this device, you run the risk of impeding the normal birthing progression.

I recommend that you have multiple opinions regarding your diagnosis and this form of treatment. I've never seen a study comparing these devices with spinal manipulation, acupuncture, massage, and exercise. I have seen it compared to exercises alone, and exercises proved to be more effective.

Are there any other mechanical aids to for the relief of back pain?

There are several products on the market that you can consider to help with the stabilization of your back when you are pregnant.

Pregnancy pillows: There are many types of these pillows on the market. They are typically five feet long, usually down filled, and tube shaped. They cost anywhere from $50.00 to $180.00. They are used to sleep with for support of your growing front side. These pillows help keep the spine from rotating while sleeping on your side.

Good walking shoes: You may have lots of shoes in your closet, but you need these for walking, not style. I recommend the kind of shoes that experienced runners use. Walking is great exercise for expectant moms, so the right shoes are crucial. These shoes need to be light (preferably not all leather) and have cool shock absorbers in them. This style of shoe will help prevent compression of the spine, knees, and hips. They should also help you avoid foot pain and fallen arches.

New bras: Due to rapid changes in breast size you will need good-fitting bras to help with midback stiffness and pain. Make sure you get fitted by someone who is experienced with maternity bras.

Maternity braces: This is a brace that fits over the abdomen in the second and third trimesters for support of the baby. This helps to disperse weight through the lower back.

These braces I find helpful for the working mothers whose backs need to be weight bearing for hours at a time. I caution not to lean on these braces late in your pregnancy. We want the baby to react to gravity and to move down into the pelvis. If overused, these types of braces may affect this transition. You also need the muscles and ligaments to slowly accommodate for the growing baby. Use these braces with caution and common sense.

Mattresses: A good mattress is worth its weight in gold when you are pregnant. I sleep on and recommend solid latex mattresses. Solid latex mattresses are not space foam or some kind of topper on a spring mattress, but a solid mix between rubber and foam. They provide great support without pressure points. These mattresses are very heavy and come in different densities. I always recommend the firmest.

CHAPTER 5

YOUR NECK AND HEADACHES (PART 1)

How can a baby in my belly hurt my neck and head?

For most women, the lower back is the major sore spot in the spinal column resulting from pregnancy. With this chapter, though, we're going to go a couple of feet higher. A significant percentage of women will go through pregnancy with little to moderate lower-back pain but will experience blasting headaches with upper-neck pain.

Since your head and your neck are fairly far removed from the load-bearing lower back, which is trying to compensate for the baby's mass and your changing center of gravity, a mechanical cause for the pain is not often diagnosed. Frequently, an ob-gyn will chalk up headaches and neck pain to hormones and recommend that you take a couple of Tylenol.

It's true that hormones can sometimes cause an imbalance that will trigger a headache. It has been my experience, however, that, more often than not, there's a mechanical cause. Chiropractors have a lot in common with car mechanics in diagnosing a condition. You hear a funny noise coming from under the hood, and a good mechanic will look for the loose doohickey or worn whatchamacallit.

Before we accept hormones as a cause, a chiropractor will determine where your pain is originating. If you have any experience with headaches, you know that sinus headaches occur in a different area of your head than a tension headache. A migraine impacts you differently than a hormonal headache.

Headaches can be brought on by mechanical interference. At this point in the discussion, many of my patients have argued, "The baby's down here," pointing to their belly. "How can it possibly affect my neck?"

I'm glad you asked. Most women who come to me with neck pain and headaches suffered from morning sickness.

How can morning sickness cause neck pain and headaches?

Nine out of ten women who come to me with headaches during pregnancy suffer from morning sickness. You're thinking that I've finally lost it, insisting that your head is somehow connected to your stomach.

Nine out of ten women who come to me with headaches during pregnancy suffer from morning sickness.

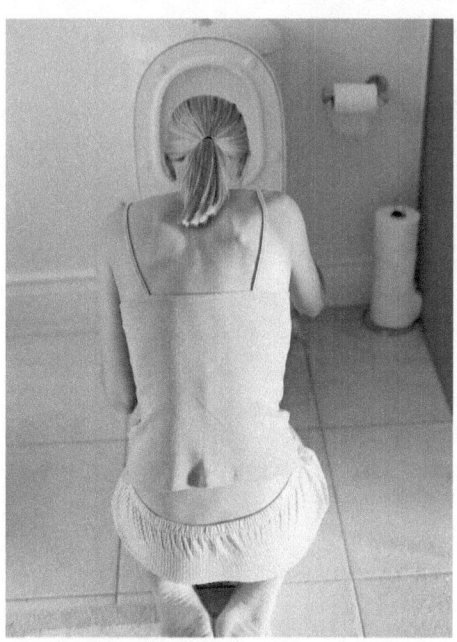

Okay, I may be nuts, but consider this: anyone who has thrown up multiple times runs the risk of neck trauma. Think through the whole process. Vomiting is a gut-wrenching, head-pounding, body-jarring event. And the part of the body where all of the action takes place isn't in your stomach; it's in your throat, which passes through the area that connects your head to your shoulders—your neck.

Not convinced? Studies have suggested that many people have herniated discs in their necks as a result of something as seemingly innocuous as sneezing. How much more violent is vomiting? How many times a week do you typically vomit with morning sickness? Only one of those events is necessary to cause a mechanical problem that will result in headache or neck pain.

How can you relieve neck pain and headaches caused by morning sickness?

Chiropractic care, combined with massage therapy, can reduce headache and neck pain caused by your bouts of morning sickness.

The mechanical problems begin with the physical act of throwing up. This creates muscle spasms over the upper back, neck, and head—including the jaw. These muscle spasms can pull or rotate some of the bones in your neck and upper back, shifting them out of place. These misaligned bones, in turn, cause symptoms like headaches, neck pain, and upper-back pain.

Your chiropractor is specifically trained to locate these misaligned vertebrae (bones) and put them back in place. The massage therapist will work to loosen the spasmodic muscles to help make sure your neck alignment isn't compromised.

CHAPTER 6

YOUR POSTURE

What does posture have to do with pregnancy?

Because the curvature of your spine will change and the weight of your baby will alter your center of gravity, pregnancy creates a major challenge for your body to maintain good posture. The changes in your body will impact the way you stand, sit, and walk. Posture becomes critical to your comfort. If you haven't discovered it yet, you may soon learn that bad posture usually leads to back pain.

First, let's define proper posture. In my world, posture is having and maintaining a *straight or erect spinal column.* My dad used to say, "Position in life is everything." He was talking about career advancement, of course; but the phrase works just as well with the way we position our spinal column when we stand, sit, and walk.

Good posture is a cosmetically acceptable stance that doesn't require expending much energy or experiencing discomfort while at rest. A traditional model for posture is to align your ear, shoulder, hip, and ankle all in the same vertical plane—on the same line, up and down.

A soldier might stand very straight while at *attention*, but he or she is burning up significant energy, stressing his or her back and neck muscles to maintain that rigid position. A soldier at attention wouldn't fit my definition of good posture because he or she has to try too hard to achieve the position.

Instead, good posture is a normal resting stance when the ligaments of the body that carry the burden of our weight are functioning economically. In other words, sitting or standing the way your body was designed with little effort.

Pregnancy complicates proper posture because, among other challenges, your ligaments are "hormonally loosened." That means your muscles have to make up for the work the ligaments would normally do in holding your body upright or in proper posture.

Your muscles have to make up for the work the ligaments would normally do in holding your body upright or in proper posture.

The work the muscles are asked to do is compromised further because there must be coordination between the muscles and the ligaments. The body is designed to send messages through the spinal cord to the brain. When you're pregnant, though, sometimes, there is some miscommunication. This is because, unlike everything else about your body that is basically symmetrical, your baby's mass is lopsided; and its weight is unevenly distributed. In addition, your baby grows quickly, especially in the third trimester. If that wasn't enough, the little darling also changes position frequently.

What happens when your baby throws your center of gravity out of whack?

Miscommunication results from the ever-changing weight imbalances you are experiencing with your baby. These weight imbalances bombard the spinal cord with *proprioception* from joints, muscles, and organs. Proprioception is the medical term that refers to the sensory experience of movements, pressure variants, and touch.

This deluge of continually changing information combined with the *righting reflex* we all have to coordinate the position of our head and eyes influences the perceived center of gravity that is impressed on the cortex or high brain to interpret the sensation of correct posture.

It's as though, for decades, your body has been communicating with your brain; and all of a sudden, it starts talking with a funny accent.

It's as though, for decades, your body has been communicating with your brain;, and all of a sudden, it starts talking with a funny accent. Information is flowing, but because it's confused, your body is reacting incorrectly.

How does posture work?

We've already established that your spinal column was designed to bend to accommodate movement.

Your body regulates posture by responding to any pressures sensed by the spinal column. When new demands are felt, the spine coordinates with the brain to change the curves of the spinal column.

As your baby grows, the curves of your spine will continue to change to accommodate its size, shape, and movement until the ligaments are stressed to the maximum. At that point, you could start to experience discomfort.

As your baby grows, the curves of your spine will continue to change to accommodate its size, shape, and movement until the ligaments are stressed to the maximum.

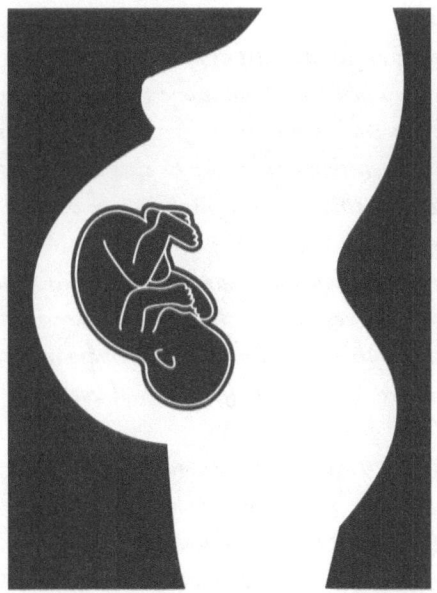

Overstretching of the ligaments will trigger and recruit a variety of muscles to maintain your optimum posture. With your muscles involved, you can expect that pain may occur, and you will also expend energy more quickly. The result could be that you'll feel both tired and achy. Sound familiar?

Appendix B in the back of this book gives you greater detail about *the anatomy of posture.*

STANDING TALL

In writing this chapter on posture, one particular patient came to mind: Sue. Sue is a patient who will follow her doctor's orders to the letter.

I remember Sue coming to me with many questions about her new pregnancy. I first saw her in her ninth week of her first pregnancy. She was in good physical shape and had been recommended to my office by one of her friends. Although Sue was never a chiropractic patient previously, she was interested in learning how to take care of her pregnant body.

First, I was amazed at the energy she had at this time in her pregnancy. It was obvious by her vigor and history she understood nutrition. I explained how her posture would behave and how it is challenging even for a woman in good shape. I recommended some stretches and activities for her to maintain good muscle tone.

One question she had was, "How often do I have to see you?" This was an excellent question.

I told her, "Generally speaking, just as often as you would see your obstetrician. At first, I see you once a month. And as we move through your pregnancy, we shorten our time frames and see each other more frequently." (This schedule is usually appropriate, especially when there are other health care practitioners involved.)

I added the caveat that this rule of thumb can go out the window if her health or environment change drastically.

Sue was a wonderful patient. She soaked up all information I gave her. She had massage work, and the result was that her posture was good throughout her pregnancy. She had no troubles at all with her framework, and her checkups were like clockwork. I explained to Sue that if I checked her spine and didn't make any corrections, she was doing great.

This was the case with Sue. She was great about diet, massage, activities, chiropractic; and her posture was a testament to her hard work. When the big event came, she had a nearly flawless labor and delivery.

Her new daughter, Megan, is just beautiful (a real doll). Megan had a good birth weight with no troubles at all. I am thankful to mothers for letting me play even a small role in the birth of their children.

How can I maintain good posture through my pregnancy?

Part of the solution to the posture challenge in pregnancy comes from the members of your health care team. In most cases, you need passive intervention. Your body needs to be stretched, strengthened, moved, touched, kneaded, and treated.

Your team needs to alter and coordinate the proprioceptive receptor signals governing your spine. Using their skills, they will essentially *reboot* your receptor-to-posture mechanism so your upper motor neurons (brain) can accept your signals of shifts in your center of gravity that will initiate appropriate alterations to the curves in your spine.

Your body needs to be stretched, strengthened, moved, touched, kneaded, and treated.

Because these members of your team work with skeletal muscles and connective tissues in different ways, they can each play a role in helping your back compensate for your pregnancy:

1. **Your massage therapist.** Getting the muscles and ligaments passively worked while in a prone position is one of the best ways to allow downtime for the brain to receive new information about the pressures on your spine. In effect, you'll trick your body into changing its neurologic firing to accept your new reality.
2. **Your acupuncturist.** Working with energy and your nervous system, acupuncture among many things will help your body accept a new reality of posture. This therapy may be longer lasting due to stimulation time of the muscles and ligaments.
3. **Your chiropractor.** Working specifically with the spinal column where most of the input is exchanged, your chiropractor will essentially recalibrate the joints and surrounding muscles and ligaments by realigning the spinal column.
4. **Your physical therapist.** By starting a stretching program or low-impact strengthening program recommended by your physical therapist, you will start firing more receptors in your body so your brain and spine can better calibrate what's happening with your body.

5. **The baby's dad.** Finally, something for that guy to do! Touch is a significant factor when dealing with the spinal column's impact on posture. Your partner needs to diligently and effectively stimulate the largest organ in your body—your skin. This will require him to do things like apply lotion to your back and legs. He'll need to rub your feet. He'll have to do whatever he can to refresh your stimuli receptors and start sending renewed signals to your brain. His concentrated touch is a process that you can experience on a daily basis to clear out all of the confusing signals your brain has had to deal with throughout your day and to update your center of gravity database.

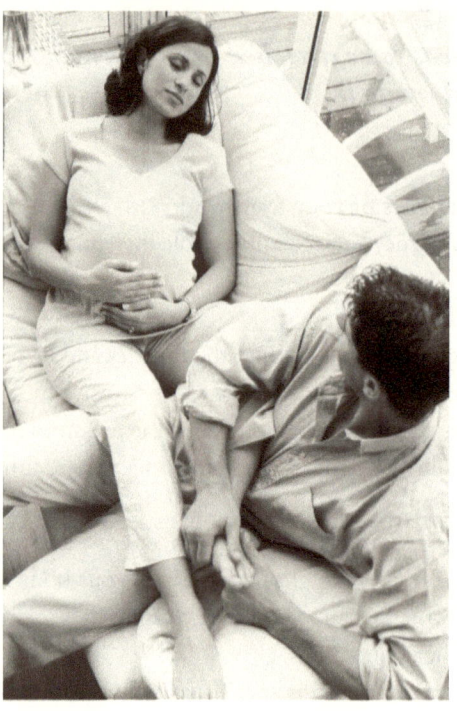

CHAPTER 7

GETTING YOURSELF IN SHAPE FOR THE BIG EVENT

What can I do to get my body ready for labor and delivery?

If they're truly honest with themselves, most women will admit they aren't in great physical shape for the ordeal their body is about to experience when they learn that they are pregnant. It's time for a little self-assessment. I need for you to evaluate your established exercise routine—not the one you were planning to start someday soon, but what you actually do now. Please check one.

☐   I exercise every day, and I'm in great shape.
☐   I exercise at least three times a week, and I'm happy with my muscle tone.
☐   I work out when I can.
☐   I prefer not to answer this question.

As we discussed in an earlier chapter, it's best to bring in some experts for help with your physical conditioning. Any member of your health care team will be able to offer you some names of physical therapists or personal athletic trainers he or she would recommend. Regardless of your current exercise routine, you should consult with a trained individual. Especially if you have an undefined workout regimen, it's critical that you get some help.

Don't be intimidated by the process. Learn how to exercise for your own benefit and for the good of your baby.

Some general guidelines to observe are the following:

1. **Check with your primary health care professional.** This is probably your ob-gyn. Make sure you don't have any complicating issues with your pregnancy that would impede or impact certain workout activities.

    A good physical therapist is going to ask whether you are cleared by your doctor, so you might as well have that answer covered before your appointment.

2. **Stay away from dangerous exercises or activities.** Few women will take up boxing or bronco busting while pregnant, but I'm often surprised by what some moms-to-be think are fine, safe pursuits in their condition. Check with your doctor.

    I always say that you can't stop a bowler from bowling or a runner from running or a horsy person from riding off into the sunset. All I can do is urge you to use caution and to keep moderation in mind at all times.

3. **Modify your activities for nine months.** Your body is going to go through many changes that will leave you susceptible to ligament and/or muscle damage. Hormonal changes alone can compromise the muscles and ligaments you've come to rely on. Even if you're a world-class athlete, you don't have the same body you had just a few months ago.

Your body is going to go through many changes that will leave you susceptible to ligament and/or muscle damage.

---

4. **Drink, drink, drink—water.** As a pregnant woman, you're more vulnerable than normal to dehydration when you participate in any sort of physical activity. Lack of fluids can lead to an elevated body temperature and uterine contractions, neither of which is good.

    When you're working out, you need to hydrate continually. If your cheeks are red and rosy after exercising, it won't be the proverbial "glow" of pregnancy; it will indicate that you're dehydrated.

    I'm a bit obsessive when it comes to water. I believe you should drink a twelve-ounce bottle of room temperature water before you exercise and another twelve-ounce bottle for each half hour of activity, regardless of how strenuous. When you're done, have another bottle. If it's hot and humid, drink even more!

When I ask expectant moms if they're drinking enough water, they always *believe* they're glugging down plenty. One pregnant patient responded, "If I pour any more water down my throat, I'll qualify as *lakefront property*."

Check your water intake, and make sure your ob-gyn is aware of what's happening with your body.

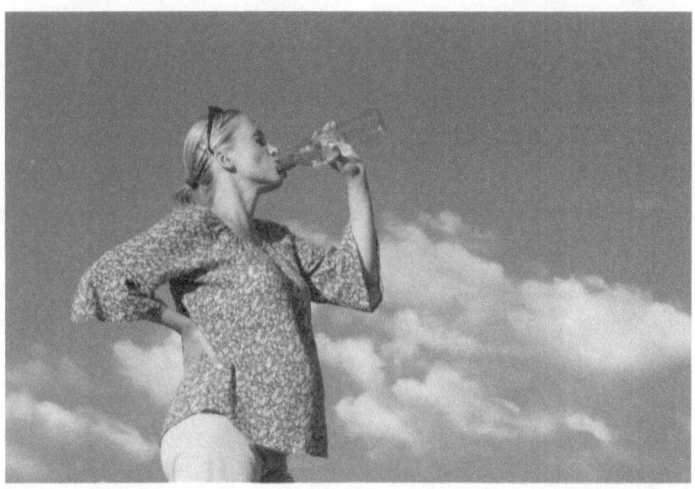

5. **Avoid getting overheated.** Please wear proper clothes when working out to help alleviate the risk of overheating. Especially when the temperatures rise, don't shroud your pregnant body. Be proud of it. Wear cool loose-fitting clothes of natural fibers like cotton.

    If you sense dizziness or if you feel flush or warm to the touch, *stop* whatever you're doing and cool down.

If you sense dizziness or if you feel flush or warm to the touch, **stop** *whatever you're doing, and cool down.*

My wife had two August babies (hey, it's cold in Colorado in December, okay?), and I got sweaty just watching her walk out to the car.

Fortunately, compared with what your mom had to wear, today's clothes are designed better and offer better fabrics to keep you modest, and cool at the same time.

6. **Eat more.** Yes, you read that correctly, eat more. Our culture has you freaking out because you're getting bigger, but that's the whole idea. You're burning calories with exercise *and* you're nourishing your baby.

   You especially need to keep your calories up when you exercise often. And remember that quality is just as important as quantity. If you don't plan on feeding your baby fries and a chocolate shake after his or her birth, why would you do it now?

   To keep your glucose levels up, you should also have a snack such as fruit or yogurt after you have completed your workout.

   According to the American Pregnancy Association, a good rule of thumb is three hundred extra calories of wholesome food daily with moderate exercise.

7. **Don't overexercise.** If you can carry on a conversation while you're working out, you aren't excessively exerting yourself. If you can't talk, you're pushing too hard—slow down or stop completely, and reevaluate your activity. If you don't have a workout partner, just talk to yourself. Just tell people you're not nuts—you're pregnant. Trust me, they'll understand.

   If you find yourself getting short of breath, take a break.

   I find it's usually in the first trimester when women overdo exercise.

There are two reasons for this phenomenon:

   a.   They are trying to hurry to get in shape.
   b.   They aren't *showing* enough to be reminded that they need to use moderation.

   You need to understand that the first trimester is critical to the development of your baby. Your body is doing extra work to make that beautiful little boy or girl. When you are *pushing it*, you're actually overexerting your developing baby too. If you're tired, take a nap. Doctor's orders!

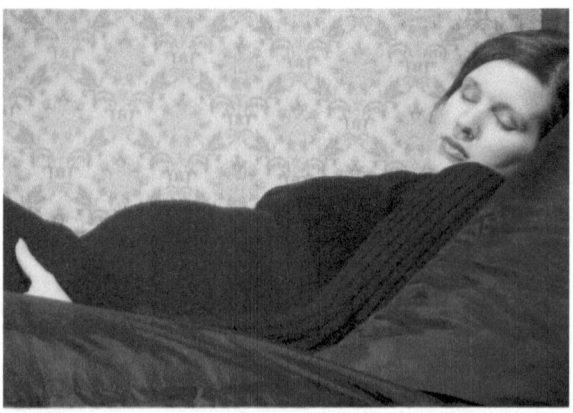

8. **Warm up and cool down properly when exercising.** Start slowly each time you work out. The warm-up can be just as beneficial as the actual workout session.

    Stretching and breathing prior to starting your exercise regimen can help increase O_2 (oxygen) to the lungs and muscles and can help you relax, preparing your body and mind. Put some love into your warm-up, and increase the effectiveness of the workout.

9. **Don't lie on your back.** There's a reason the back of the table props up in your doctor's office and why the nurse will put a pillow behind your back.

    If you lie flat on your back for a few minutes or more during the later months of the pregnancy (after about twenty-fourth week), you may start to feel light-headed, dizzy, and possibly breathless. That's because your growing baby is putting pressure on one of your major blood vessels called the *vena cava*. The vena cava lies on the right side of your body. During pregnancy, your enlarged uterus also naturally leans toward your right side (as it moves up and out of the pelvis after twelve weeks). This can make the vena cava blood vessel prone to becoming compressed while lying on your back. Learn to lie on your side, preferably your left side, so you uterus is moved away from your vena cava.

10. **Include the dad whenever possible.** Pregnancy isn't an individual sport. It took two of you to get into this condition, and getting out of it is best when it's a team event.

    I always urge dads to get involved with your walks or other physical activities a couple of times a week over all forty weeks. Every coach your significant other has ever heard of goes to all of the practices and workouts. There's no coach around who would ever think to just show up on *game day* for the main event. It's a terrific opportunity to share communication and motivation.

I always urge dads to get involved with your walks or other physical activities a couple of times a week over all forty weeks.

---

11. **Listen to your body.** Pace yourself. If you work a full eight-hour day, adapt your workouts. If need be, some days, just limit your activity to your stretches if that's what your body is telling you.

    If your body tells you to stop exercising completely, though, you probably misunderstood. Ask it to repeat itself and listen more carefully. Rest now and then, but keep working out for your own good and for the good of your baby.

12. **Stretch before working out.** Slow, steady stretching will help muscles stay loose and flexible. This is important at all times, but especially when you're pregnant. Along with improving flexibility, stretching will allow your body to relax and unwind after a tough day while warming up your muscles. Stretching again at the end of your workout will also improve your flexibility.

13. **Watch for swelling.** This is also known as *edema* (sometimes known as *dropsy* or *hydropsy*). Edema is the increase of interstitial fluid in any organ. For example, if you notice swelling of your ankles or fingers that lasts after you've finished cooling down at the end of your workout, you'll need to make some modifications to your regimen.

    What are obvious signs of swelling? Your rings are too tight, or your socks leave an indentation around your ankle. As soon as you get home after any sort of workout, elevate your feet.

    If the expectant dad is available, put him to work rubbing your feet to flush pooling blood. Give him the "It's for the baby" routine. It works every time in my house.

CHAPTER 8

YOUR STRETCHES

Does the world really need another book on stretches?

No. That's why this chapter is brief and more obligatory for me to include than mandatory for you to follow. I'm realistic enough to realize that if you haven't been doing stretches before you got pregnant, chances are slim that you'll start now.

Of course, I encourage them.

While researching this book, I discovered that there are already a tremendous number of books specifically about lower-back stretches and pregnancy. There were also multiple books on yoga and pregnancy as well as pilates and pregnancy and even belly dancing and pregnancy.

Workouts for pregnancy come in book form as well as videos. There's another whole bookshelf of celebrities preaching perfect ways for pregnant women to get in shape.

A Google search of "stretches for pregnant women" results in nearly 1.2 million hits. "Exercises during pregnancy" gives you about 1.4 million hits.

I'm sure that most of these books, videos, and Web sites have merit. I asked my wife, Gina, what she thought of the books on the market that she had read when she was pregnant. She endorsed virtually every one of them, and then she burst the bubble. "When," she asked, "is a pregnant woman today going to find even an hour a day three times a week to devote to stretching?"

She's right. The book can be excellent, but if all you do is read it and don't actually follow its advice, you're not accomplishing anything.

In the real world, women work eight hours a day throughout their pregnancy, and many have children already at home who need love and attention. It's tough enough to get through the day and find time for a shower, let alone workout time.

Early in my practice, after correcting an expectant mother's spine, I would give her sheets of paper with stretches diagrammed for them. I would spend the time explaining the stretches and their importance. Often, we would be encircled by the mom's brood of toddlers and young children.

What was I thinking? The printed sheets of stretches might have made it all the way to the floorboard of the car or maybe ended up attached to the refrigerator with a magnet, never to be looked at again. It was unreasonable of me to think that my patients could take my stretching-exercise lecture seriously. There simply wasn't enough time or energy left in the day to get into a regular routine. Life was getting in the way of my grand plan.

Don't get me wrong. Stretches are important, and I urge all of my patients to do them religiously. I've simply had enough clinical experience to know that we're fighting an uphill battle. That's why, when necessary, I have included things like massage therapy, physical therapy, and acupuncture to my chiropractic treatment of expectant moms.

Massage therapy can be an excellent alternative to stretches in many ways. It's passive—you don't do any of the work; just show up and lie down with your eyes closed. And you still get your muscles worked and stretched.

Why are stretches important to protect my back?

If you can find the time, stretches are a valuable tool for keeping your back pain free. By repeatedly taking your muscles to tension and releasing them, you break down a small amount of connective tissue so they can be rebuilt to produce greater flexibility and strength.

Athletes stretch before they perform so they don't "pull a hammy," their hamstring or other muscle group. Pregnant women stretch to help maintain proper receptor input from the connective tissue to their central nervous system. The result should be improved posture and reduced chance of back pain.

Pregnant women stretch to help maintain proper receptor input from the connective tissue to their central nervous system.

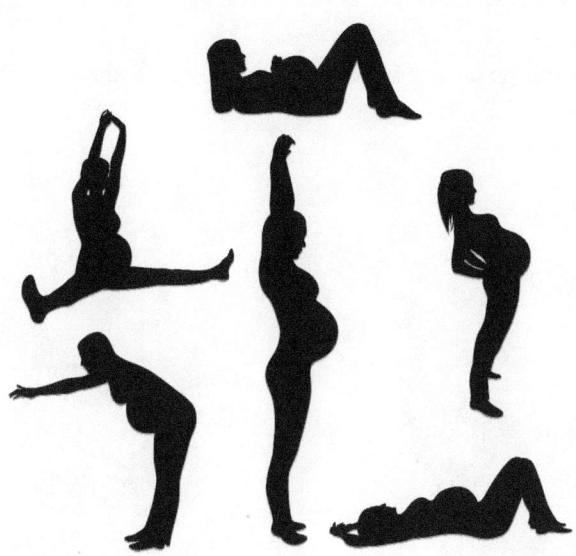

Stretching and breathing go hand in hand. Any time I can encourage an expectant mother to breathe deeply for an extended period of time, I have seen that there are benefits for both the mom *and* her baby.

Not all stretches are created equal. Most might be great for many women, but perhaps not for you. Don't do anything you find uncomfortable or awkward. Our goal is to prevent injury, not cause it.

Before you start stretching, visit your chiropractor, and make sure you don't have any preexisting condition that would preclude any specific physical activities in your pregnant condition. And always check with your ob-gyn to make sure you're cleared for any physical activities outside your daily routine.

The following are a few stretches that I recommend for most pregnant patients. I will explain potential pitfalls with some of the specific movements.

UPPER-BACK AND NECK STRETCHES

Wall press. The purpose of this movement is to stretch the upper back, neck, and chest.

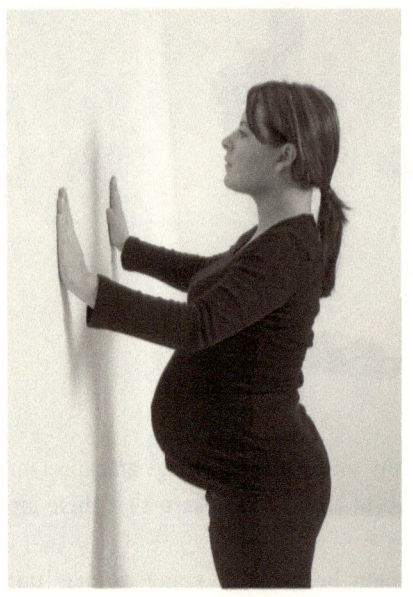 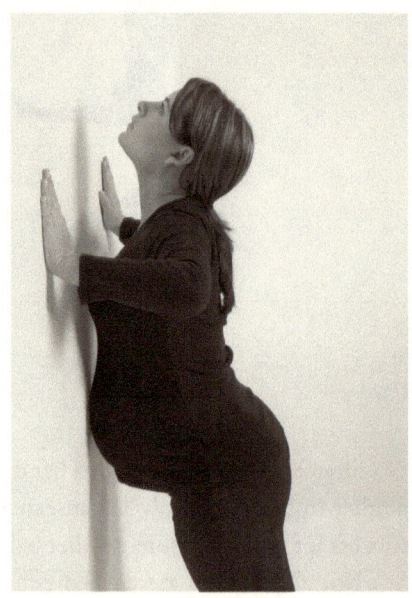

1. Start by standing at arm's length from the wall.
2. Place both hands on the wall at shoulder height.
3. Squeeze your shoulder blades together and down.
4. Slowly bend arms, and touch your nose to the wall. Keep your spine straight and your neck at a slight extension.
5. From this position, push your shoulder blades apart, tuck in your chin, and push your midback away from the wall.
6. Hold for ten seconds, and then return to the starting position.
7. Repeat the entire sequence five times.

Pectoral major and minor stretch. The purpose of this is to stretch the chest and shoulders.

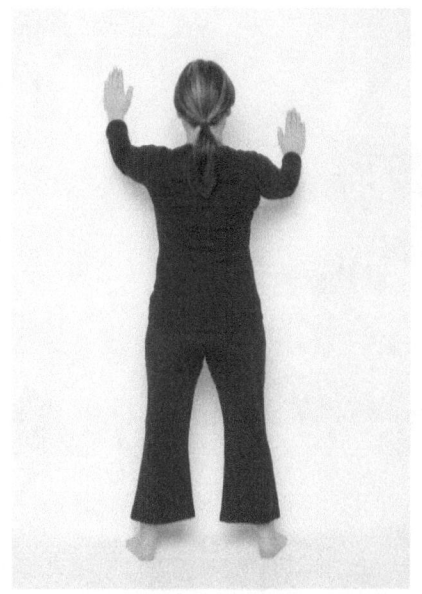 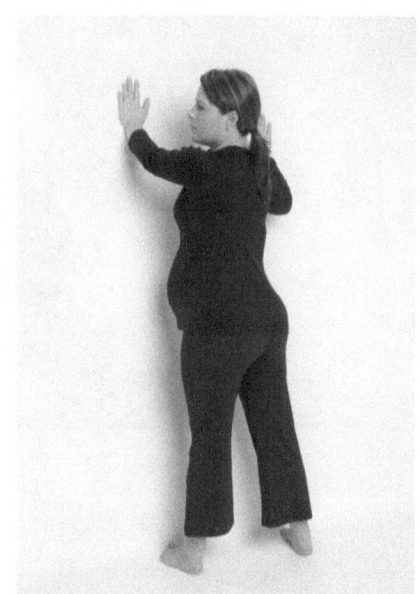

Don't arch your back during this exercise.
1. Start by facing the wall.
2. Reach your right hand straight out from your shoulder against the wall just below shoulder height.
3. Place your left hand firmly on the wall at chin height.
4. Bend your left elbow down to bring your right shoulder blade down and back.
5. Maintain this position so your feet are perpendicular to the wall.
6. Press your right fingertips against the wall to help turn your chest to the right.
7. Slowly turn your chest around to the right, opening both sides of your chest and feeling a stretch in the front of the right shoulder and chest.

Don't allow your right shoulder to elevate during the stretch.
8. Hold for ten seconds.
9. Repeat five times.
10. Repeat with the left side five times.

Serratus anterior stretch. The purpose of this stretch is to strengthen you from your shoulder girdle to your spine. This will help with upper-back strength and breast-feeding after the baby is born.

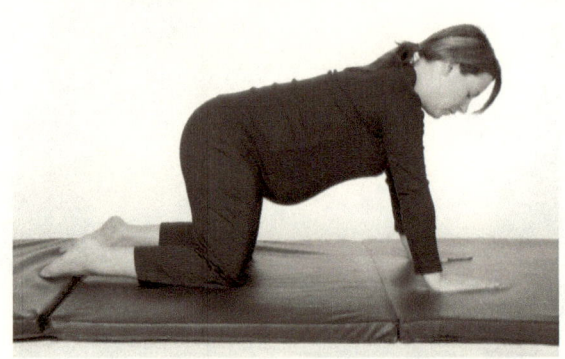

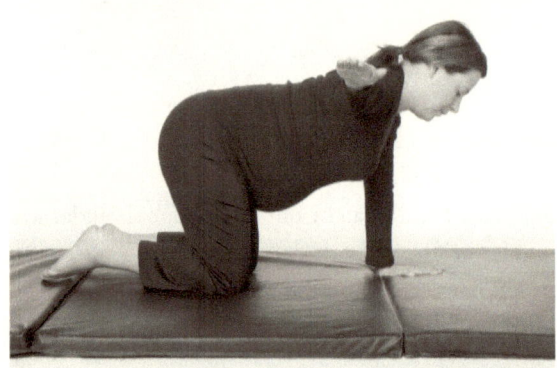

1. Begin on your hands and your knees, with your hips over your knees and your shoulders over your hands.
2. Press your midback up toward the ceiling and tuck your chin in.
3. Hold for ten seconds.
4. While maintaining this position, lift your left hand off the floor and to the side.
5. Hold for ten seconds.
6. Relax for five to ten seconds.
7. Repeat using the opposite hand.
8. Do each hand a total of five times.

Lower trapezius training. The purpose of this stretch is to strengthen your shoulder girdle and midback. This will help keep your shoulders pulled back later in your pregnancy. The position of this stretch makes it particularly beneficial in early pregnancy.

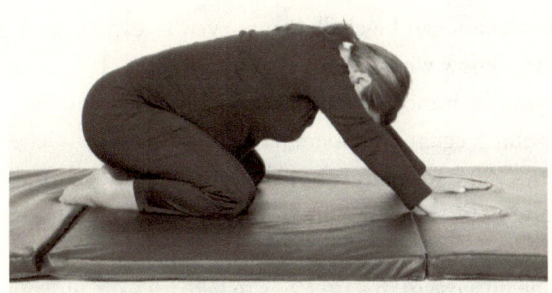

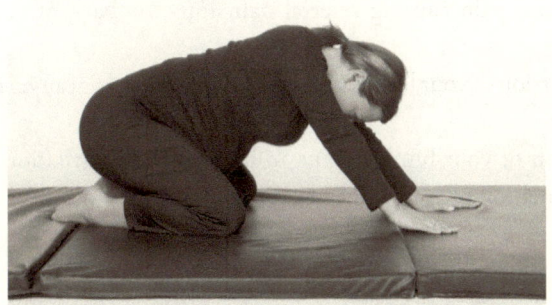

This will be a difficult exercise to perform after your twentieth week.

1. Begin on your hands and knees.
2. Sit back on your heels and bend forward with your forehead toward the floor
3. Pull your shoulder blades down and back. Do not squeeze your shoulder blades together.
4. Hold for ten seconds.
5. Repeat five times both sides.

LOWER-BACK STRETCHES

Not all stretches targeting the lower back are beneficial. It is important to understand what is happening in your lower back and what stresses and strains it is under.

As I have mentioned in previous chapters, there are two common types of lower-back pain. Discerning which type of pain you have is important before any exercise or stretch over the lower back and pelvis.

Diagnosing back pain can be challenging, even to experienced diagnosticians, so don't assume that you know where your pain is originating. If you get advice from your best girlfriend or your own mother (trust me, you will) on how she got rid of pain in her lower back during pregnancy, remember that her pain may have been completely different from yours. All back pain is not the same, even when the symptoms sound similar. Get a second opinion, preferably from a health care professional.

Cat and camel. The purpose of this stretch is to take pressure off your spine and gently stretch your lower back. This is a standard stretch for expectant moms because it is good for a wide variety of lower-back conditions such as the following:

1. Nerve root pain causing referral pain into the back of your buttocks and thighs
2. Compression of your lumbosacral plexus in your pelvis caused by your enlarging uterus
3. Extension of your lumbar spine to help with disc irritation or symptomatic disc herniation of your spine

Breathing is very important with this stretch.

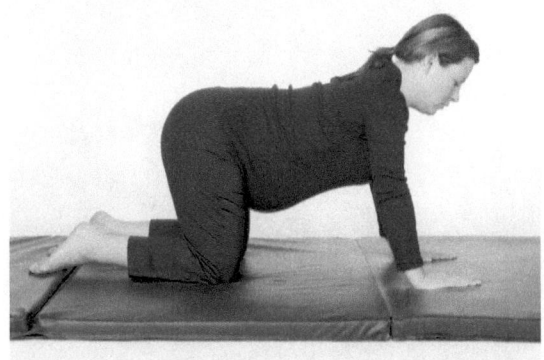

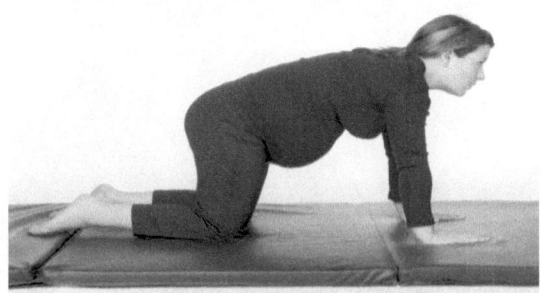

1. Start on your hands and knees, with your shoulders vertically above your wrists and with your hips above your knees.
2. On an inhaled breath, arch your back upward while lowering your head. Try to round your spine as much as comfortably possible.
3. Without changing your position, tuck your pelvis under, using your abdominals and buttocks.
4. Hold for five seconds.
5. When you exhale, lift your head upward, and push your chest and abdomen toward the floor.
6. Hold for five seconds.
7. Repeat steps 2 through 6 five times.

Prayer stretch. The purpose of this stretch is twofold: (1) to allow for extension of your lumbar spine as in the cat and camel and (2) to gently stretch your lumbar to pelvic muscle attachments without flexion of your trunk.

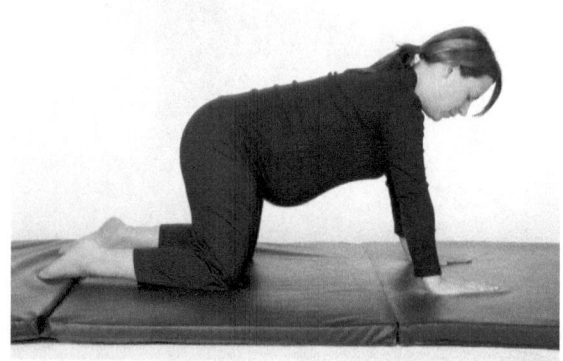

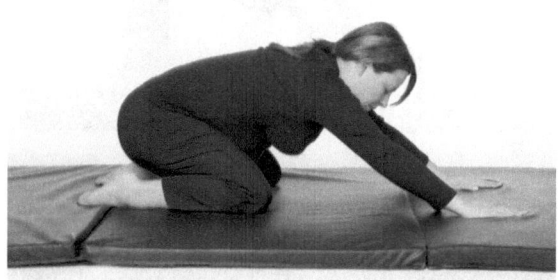

1. Start on your hands and knees, with your arms stretched out in front of you.
2. Extend your hips backward and move your face close to the floor, trying to touch your buttocks to your heels.
3. Hold for ten seconds.
4. Return to the starting position.
5. Repeat previous steps five times.

Kneeling stretch. The purpose of this stretch is to laterally stretch your lower back, pelvis, and hips without flexion of your trunk.

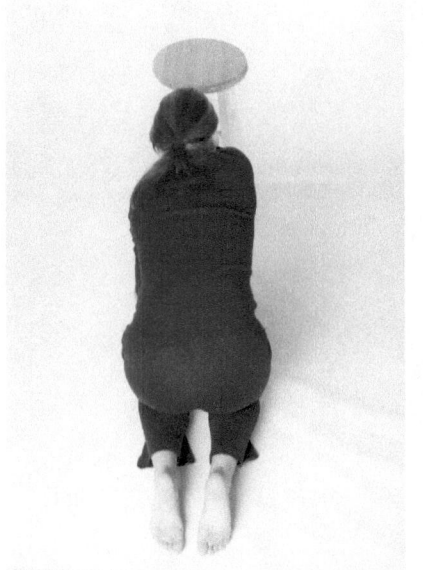 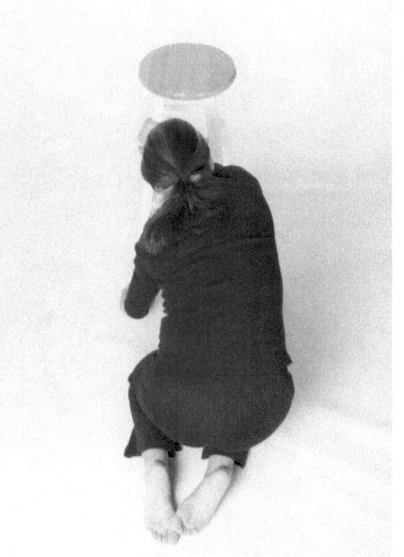

1. Start in the hands-and-knees position.
2. Reach forward with your right hand, and grasp a secure object, such as a doorjamb or stool.
3. From this position, sit back diagonally toward the right buttocks, elongating the right side.
4. The right arm may be internally rotated to increase the stretch.
5. Work on elongation of the right side by dropping the pelvis further diagonally backward and toward the hip.
6. Hold for ten seconds.
7. Repeat on the opposite side.
8. Repeat for a total of five cycles on each side.

Pelvic tilt. The purpose of this stretch is to strengthen abdominal and internal hip flexors. Keep your lower back flat on the floor for this exercise up through the fourth month of pregnancy. During the final five months, this stretch can be done in a standing position with your back flat against a wall. This stretch will prepare you for the birthing process.

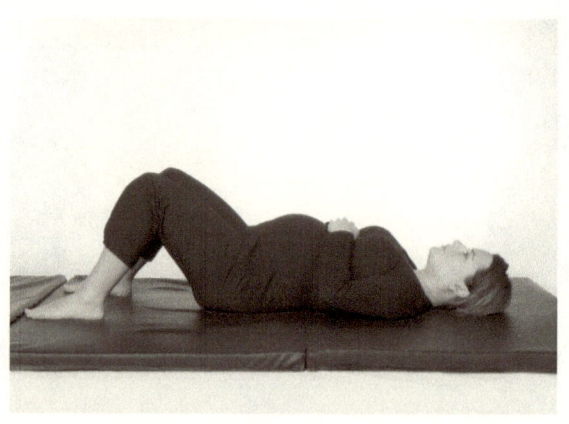

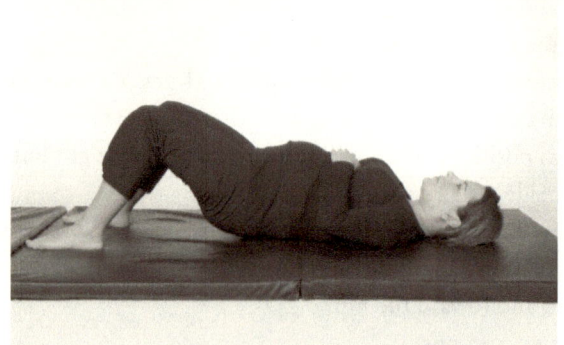

1. Begin by lying on your back with your knees bent and your feet flat on the floor.
2. Push the lower part of your back into the floor by tightening your abdominal and buttock muscles.
3. Rotate your pelvis upward without bringing your back off the floor.
4. Hold for five seconds, and then return to the starting position.
5. Relax for five seconds.
6. Repeat five times.

Breathing is important. *Do not hold your breath.*

Bridging. This stretch is great for strengthening abdominals and stabilizing your lower back.

This should not be performed past your fourth month of pregnancy.

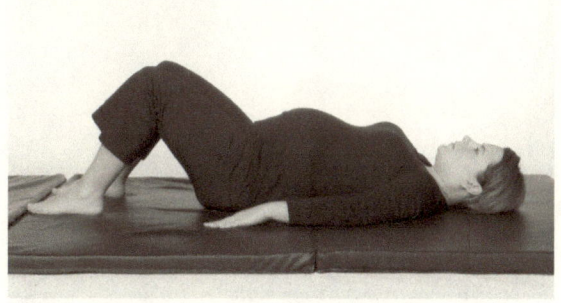

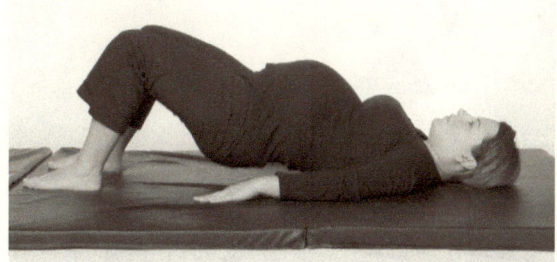

1. Begin by lying on your back, knees bent, and feet flat on the floor. Extend your arms out to the sides to steady yourself.
2. Squeeze your buttocks and raise your hips and lower back off the floor to form a straight line from your knees to your chest.

Do not arch your back.

3. Hold for five to ten seconds.
4. Slowly return to the starting position.
5. Relax for five seconds.
6. Repeat five times.
7. Stay in pain-free range.

Lateral leg splits. This is great for strengthening your hip muscles and stabilizing your lumbar spine. This can also be done by getting on all fours and lifting your thigh and leg to the side. Done on all fours, this stretch is sometimes called *fire hydrants* because when you lift your leg, it looks like a dog peeing on a fire hydrant. A male dog, of course. Go figure.

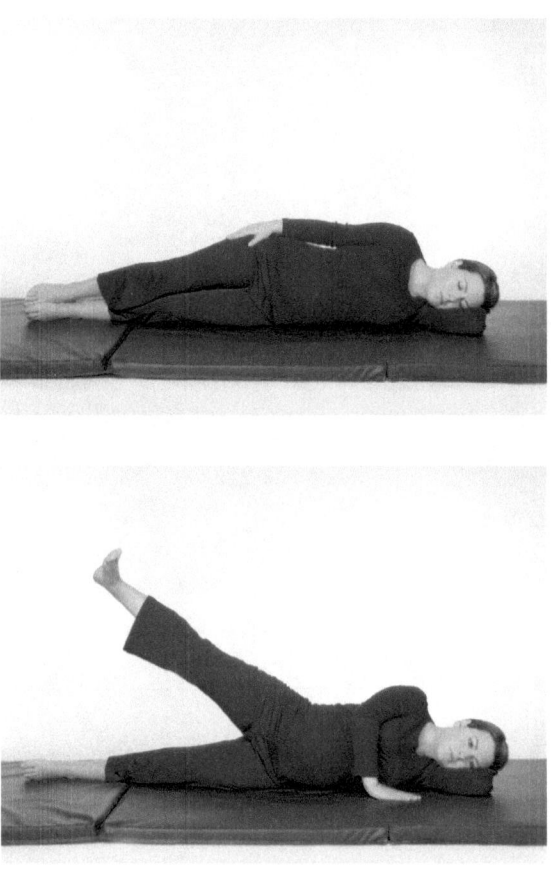

1. Lie on your left side, resting your upper body weight on your elbow.
2. Using your hand for balance, lift your right leg upward as high as is comfortably possible.
3. Hold for ten seconds.
4. Slowly lower to the starting position.
5. Repeat ten times.
6. Roll over, and repeat on your right side with your left leg.
7. Repeat ten times.

Be sure to keep your back straight.

Back builder. This is a great stretch designed to strengthen both your upper and lower back.

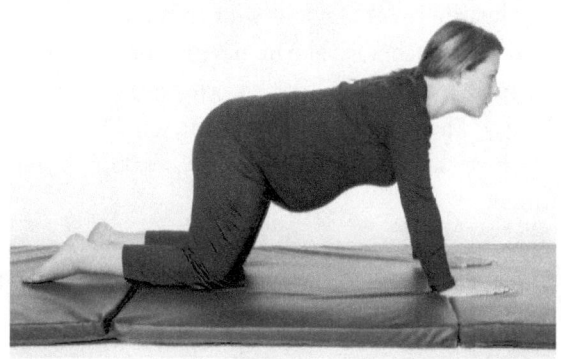

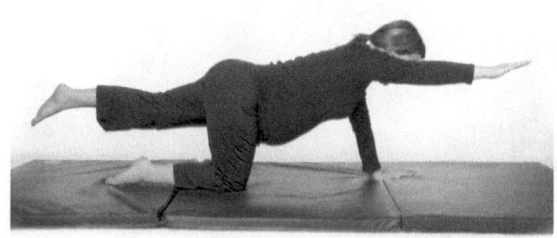

1. Begin on your hands and knees, looking down at the floor.
2. Simultaneously, raise and straighten your right arm and left leg until they are parallel to the ground.
3. Hold for ten seconds.
4. Repeat five to ten times.
5. Repeat steps 2 through 4 using your left arm and right leg.

Keep your abdominal muscles tight.
Don't sag your chest or hips.
Keep breathing. Do not hold your breath.

ADDITIONAL STRETCHES

There are far too many stretches and exercises to list every one. This is just a sampling, a starting point. All activities should be under the supervision of your appropriate health care team member, primarily your ob-gyn or your chiropractor.

What do most of the stretches listed here have in common? Most are on all fours and provide lumbar spine extension. This is to give your lumbar discs a break if you have been sitting all day. They allow you to carry the weight back on the joints where it belongs. As you get larger as your pregnancy progresses, I think you'll see the wisdom of the all fours position.

CHAPTER 9

YOUR PHYSICAL ACTIVITIES

What about specific sports and activities?

Now that the ground rules are established and you have stretched, you're probably wondering what sorts of exercises, sports, or activities you should be doing. If you're already running or swimming, for example, modify your workouts appropriately. If exercising isn't part of your normal routine, check with your doctor or physical therapist. The following are some of my opinions about the activities my patients have undertaken while pregnant.

RECOMMENDED ACTIVITIES

Walking. This is by far the preferred exercise in my practice. You can do it throughout the nine months of pregnancy and for the rest of your life. What makes walking so attractive is that it works your heart muscle, yet you can do it anywhere. It doesn't jar your knees, ankles, or spine. You can do it with another person. And you can tailor your workout to your physical condition and your pregnancy. Walking is totally adaptable. I recommend getting a good pair of walking shoes and possibly buying some arm weights to prepare your arms for baby lifting.

What makes walking so attractive is that it works your heart muscle, yet you can do it anywhere.

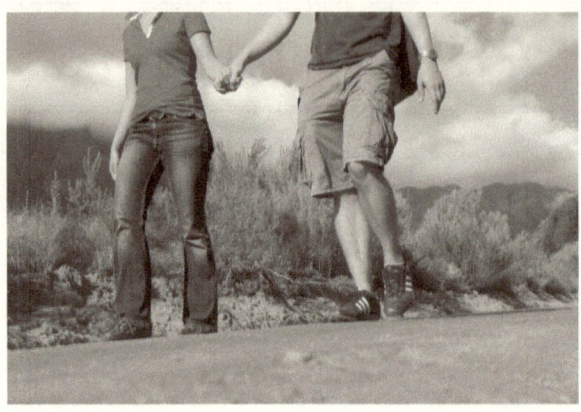

Walk briskly to get your heart rate up. In the early stages of pregnancy, I recommend that you walk for about thirty minutes or about two miles. You should taper down the length and duration of your walk as your pregnancy gets late into the second trimester and throughout the third trimester.

Also, as you get further along in your pregnancy, the place where you walk becomes important. Hiking over uneven ground starts to become a bad idea in your second trimester.

My wife and I live in Colorado, so my advice to expectant moms in higher altitudes is to go for walks of twenty to thirty minutes. This is due to the mile-high air being less rich in oxygen than the air closer to sea level.

As noted previously in chapter 7, be aware of possible contractions; and follow the warning signs listed earlier, especially swelling of the feet and ankles.

Swimming. This takes a little more preparation than walking—you have to know how to swim—but it's a great aerobic workout. Swimming is especially spine friendly because there is no bone-jarring impact, and gravity is not an issue taxing your joints and ligaments.

Swimming is also a great exercise because it uses both large and small muscle groups of both the upper and lower body. Even a gentle swim provides you with a great cardiovascular workout that boosts your circulation and aids the transportation of oxygen and nutrients around your body. This helps you to feel energized and also reduces water retention and swelling.

In addition, swimming works every major muscle group in your body, so making a regular trip to the pool will facilitate the development of muscle tone. This will help you to adapt to your changing shape and will also make it easier to regain your prepregnancy figure after you've given birth.

Swimming also begins to build endurance and endorphin responses that can make you better equipped to tolerate pain during labor.

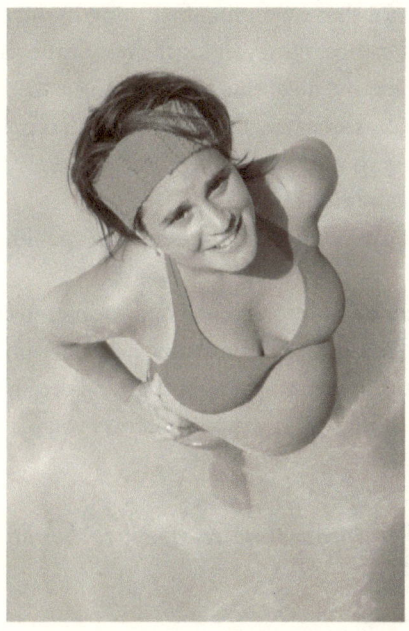

In my practice, I've noticed that swimming also begins to build endurance and endorphin responses that can make you better equipped to tolerate pain during labor.

Submersion in water provides you with a weightless environment in which to work out, so swimming poses almost no risk of joint or ligament injury and can actually help to reduce aches and pains by supporting your body as you move. This is especially beneficial during pregnancy as your joints, muscles, and ligaments become particularly susceptible to damage as increased hormone levels cause them to soften and become overly flexible.

Although exercising in the water will help to reduce the chances of overheating, it is still important to drink plenty of fluids before, during, and after you swim to prevent dehydration. Even though you don't sense that you are perspiring because of the nature of the activity, you sweat when you swim.

I encourage my patients to swim the breaststroke whenever possible because it requires no rotation of the neck, and it generally requires less exertion. The breaststroke also helps counteract the increased strain on your back due to the belly weight of pregnancy. While pregnancy forces your spine and shoulders to round forward and your pelvis to tilt out of alignment, the breaststroke gently strengthens your hip flexor muscles and counteracts that tendency. Breaststroke is particularly helpful in improving your posture and reducing backache by strengthening your abdominal, back, chest, and shoulder muscles.

If you're able, I recommend that you swim for at least thirty minutes a day. It has been my clinical experience that swimming first thing in the morning while pregnant helps control nausea and can energize you for the rest of the day.

From my point of view, the downside to swimming is that it does not prepare your spine for handling the baby's weight quite as well as walking. It is an excellent option, though, if you have access to water and if you need to be selective with your activities due to some pregnancy conditions.

Remember, when you're swimming, the blood isn't pooling in your feet.

Water walking and water aerobics. Here's an opportunity to combine the best of both walking and swimming. You don't need to know how to swim to benefit from a water workout. You can walk, jog, or even run in waist-high and deeper water to strengthen your core trunk muscles, legs, and hips. It will also increase your cardiorespiratory fitness.

You don't need to know how to swim to benefit from a water workout.

If you find traveling from one end of the pool to another boring, find a walking buddy. Or consider joining a water aerobics class for expectant moms.

Exercising in water is ideal for pregnant women because the water's buoyancy only requires you to support 50 percent of your body weight. That reduces the risk of stress-related injuries. And the compression of the water is soothing to joints and muscles that are already stressed by the added dimension of your pregnancy. As I mentioned in the swimming section, the water temperature keeps you from overheating during your workout.

You can do *stair-step* exercises on the stairs leading into the pool if there are any. That repetitive movement will strengthen your hips and upper legs.

A water walking exercise that I like to recommend is called the Charlie Chaplin walk. It specifically targets your middle and upper back. Here's what you do:

> Tuck your elbows into your sides, hold your hands out to your sides, ideally in the water, with your palms flat and your thumbs pointing up. This will create resistance as you walk. Walk the width of the pool both forward and backward.

Yoga, pilates, and tai chi. Although there isn't as much data available on pilates as yoga and tai chi, these disciplines all appear to be very effective in both stretching and strengthening. Which activity you choose will depend on your own interests and lifestyle. Do some research online, or talk to friends and relatives. Many local health clubs will offer classes for each of these disciplines.

I would caution you that if you've never done these actions, get with an instructor first. Don't keep the fact that you're pregnant a secret. You want him or her to recommend exercises that can be customized to your condition. Again, take it slow, and build up to an appropriate exercise routine. If you're already doing one of these activities, modify it for your current condition.

> **Yoga.** This is a great activity for several reasons. The first is pretty basic: yoga teaches every student to *breathe*. I know you've been breathing your whole life, but the breathing techniques you learn in yoga will help improve energy and decrease stress during the first trimester. In the third trimester, with your changed breathing mechanics, yoga will teach you to breathe more efficiently to help eliminate neck pain during the delivery of your baby while increasing your oxygen intake.
>
> Yoga breathing will also come in handy with the accompanying pains associated with labor and delivery.
>
> Many yoga exercises are quite similar to the stretches discussed in the previous chapter. I would avoid doing any yoga poses on your back or stomach, but many of the other poses are perfect for your pregnant body. You can also try to modify the back (or supine) poses by doing them on your side. You can try doing the prone poses on your knees if necessary.
>
> I recommend that you discuss your condition with your instructor to carefully modify your routine.

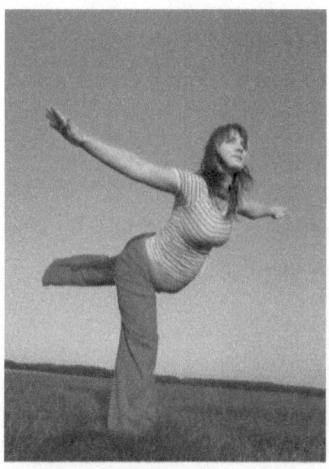

Pilates. This is also a good activity when you're pregnant because pilates is based on flowing movements—no sudden, jerky actions. Instead, one position flows as slowly and naturally as possible into the next. You move rhythmically.

You set your pace with your own breathing, and this warms the muscles and makes them lengthen out rather than bunch and bulk up. Moving slowly also gives you time to become aware of each part of your body so that you perform all the exercises with precision.

Relaxation is an important element of pilates, but especially during pregnancy when you may often be overwhelmed with feelings of tiredness. Pilates relaxation will help to restore flagging energy levels and, just as crucially, to induce a more tranquil state of mind.

Tai chi. Not chai tea, that's a popular drink in coffee shops around the country. Tai chi is actually an ancient Chinese martial art, t'ai chi ch'uan. I highly recommend this discipline to my patients, including expectant moms.

Tai chi, sometimes also called *taiji*, is often described as *moving meditation*. When you do tai chi, you use various sets of smooth movements while mimicking nature and animals. The discipline is primarily used to gently move blood and energy.

Tai chi is also very good for learning controlled breathing with many of the benefits of yoga.

(You probably noticed that I recommended acupuncture earlier in the book. Now I'm promoting tai chi. Obviously, I'm willing to go to the other side of the planet to find ways to help you minimize back pain during pregnancy. Next, *The Wonders of Moo Shu Vegetables.*)

Some benefits of yoga, pilates, and tai chi:

- builds arm and leg strength (which will help carrying your baby)
- assists with labor with deep-breathing techniques
- increases oxygen flow
- increases body awareness
- easy to learn
- uses gentle motions to tone muscles without straining
- promotes correct body posture
- improves balance
- requires no special equipment
- suitable for virtually everyone
- shown to improve blood pressure
- assists mental well-being through meditative forms

♦   improves coordination and flexibility
♦   improves relaxation

DVD workouts. I have actually seen and evaluated many very good exercise DVDs for pregnant moms. This form of exercise is one of my favorites because you can work out in the comfort and convenience of your own home, and for many moms, this is critical. Again, don't overdo it. Be aware of your limits, and work your way up to an everyday routine.

Avoid any jumping, lunging, or leaping DVDs because those activities are not recommended for women in your condition. With new DVDs coming on the market and older versions going off, it would be counterproductive to list recommended DVDs here. Probably the best bet would be to ask a friend or relative who has just given birth which video she found particularly beneficial.

I love it when my wife gathers the kids together, and they do the exercise video as a group.

ACTIVITIES TO UNDERTAKE WITH CAUTION

Low-impact aerobics. This activity is good for your heart and lungs, but must be monitored closely. I urge my patients to join a class specifically designed for mothers-to-be. The advantages to these classes are as follows:

1.   The exercises are selected for your condition.
2.   The pace is modified to your condition.
3.   You are surrounded and supported by others in your condition.
4.   Chances are there's day care available if you have other children, allowing you some "me" time.

Weight training in a gym. Unless you are already completely at ease in the weight room, I would discourage you from engaging in this form of exercise. With concerns about your joint laxity, ligament instability, heart rate, oxygen consumption, and overheating, starting a weight training program now could be very traumatic on your body. This is definitely not the kind of stress that we want to put your body through at this time.

If you are already committed to weight training, be advised that it's almost impossible to find guidelines on weight training while pregnant. I'm guessing that there aren't many proponents of pumping iron when you're pregnant.

The best I can do is recommend that you modify your program so that you are performing something like six sets of five reps each, or ten sets of three reps, for the same total volume, but reducing the demands of each set to reflect the increased need for rest and moderation.

Be advised that weight machines are not structurally designed for moms-to-be. Free weights are a safer choice. But even with dumbbells and hand weights, you are at risk for aggravating and prolonging your ligament instability.

Avoid weight training totally if you have a preexisting back condition.

ACTIVITIES TO AVOID

Bicycling. If your exercise of choice is usually bike riding, we may have an issue. Your sacroiliac and lumbosacral joints become compromised during mid to late pregnancy, and standard bicycling stresses those joints due to your flexing the trunk of your body.

I only recommend that pregnant women ride a recumbent bike, that's the low-slung two—or three-wheeler with the back—support seat and your legs parallel to the ground. With a recumbent bike, you can put pressure on the back side of the pelvis and create short controlled, nonstressing lever movements through the sacroiliac and lumbosacral joints. You also tend to use your hip flexors (thighs) more than with a standard bike. Stationary recumbent bikes are usually standard equipment at gyms and fitness centers.

As far as getting up and down off the bike while you're pregnant, you're on your own. (That may take more energy than the workout itself.)

Elliptical machine. I'm compelled to discourage you from using an elliptical machine. I don't like any of my patients using them. Ever. I'm not fond of the pedal-type stair steppers either. These machines certainly aren't designed for expectant moms.

Elliptical machines are a great source of patients for chiropractors. I'd vote to have them banned or at least require a surgeon general's warning: "Caution, use of this device is known to cause pelvic imbalance and bad posture."

Watch people on an elliptical machine. Invariably, they'll favor a dominant leg and foot. That can create an imbalance in your pelvis and contribute to bad pelvic alignment and bad posture.

Another problem I have with elliptical machines is that while your back health care team is trying to eliminate shear forces through the sacroiliac joints, the machine clearly does just the opposite, potentially causing damaging rotation of the sacroiliac joints.

If those problems weren't enough, there's also the stress you put on your joints and back ligaments leaning forward to grip the handles. Most elliptical machines are engineered to accommodate the average height of an adult in the United States—five feet ten inches. Unfortunately, the average height of a female adult in the United States is five feet four inches. That means, even when you're not pregnant, you are putting stress on your back continually while you work out by extending your reach to make up for six inches.

Also, stay away from activities such as aerobic dance, bench-step classes, kickboxing aerobics, snow-skiing, water-skiing, and roller-blading. It is crucial to choose exercises, activities, and sports that do not result in a loss of balance since a fall during this period could prove harmful or even fatal for both the mother and the baby.

It is crucial to choose exercises, activities, and sports that do not result in a loss of balance.

CHAPTER 10

YOUR PREGNANCY AND WORK

What can I do to protect my back while working during pregnancy?

Today, more than half of all American women work outside the home. If only 2 percent of the approximately fifty million women who are of childbearing age and working outside the home are expecting a baby at any given time, approximately one million working women are pregnant at this moment in the United States.

With such a large number of pregnant employees, many employers recognize the need to address workplace safety. Because of employer liability issues, the concern is usually concentrated on obvious things like chemical exposure, radiation exposure, and other readily apparent workplace hazards.

Somewhat under the radar is the fact that ergonomic concerns also exist. The very act of doing your job can create severe and lingering back pain. Ergonomics is the science of fitting the job to the worker rather than the worker to the job. When you start thinking about your job in terms of your environment and the tasks you must accomplish, it's easy to see that no matter what your job is, chances are excellent that as your baby grows, you'll no longer fit your workspace.

It's easy to see that no matter what your job is, chances are excellent that as your baby grows, you'll no longer fit your workspace.

For example, the baby growing in your uterus can affect how far you can reach, your balance, and any lifting tasks. Because your ligaments loosen during pregnancy, your condition can also aggravate the effects of repetitive motion tasks.

Not to be an alarmist, but I have read several troubling reports and studies that suggest certain work-related ergonomic stressors can lead to adverse pregnancy outcomes, such as preterm delivery, low birth weight, and, in rare cases, spontaneous abortion. Multiple studies have found an increased risk of preterm delivery among women whose jobs combine several workplace stress factors, such as standing for a long period of time, repetitive lifting, and working long hours.

In fact, my experience is that more women are at risk for a complicated back pain—intense pregnancy because of mundane everyday tasks like reaching, sitting, and standing than from our more typical fears like climbing ladders and exposure to solvents and chemicals.

Here are some concerns to consider with your pregnancy:

- awkward postures
- heavy lifting
- limited rest periods
- repetitive movements

Back pain and carpal tunnel syndrome (CTS) are both relatively common side effects of working during pregnancy, and both may be aggravated by routine job tasks.

Pregnancy alters your body's shape and, therefore, the way you adapt to your work site. As your abdomen grows, you will usually experience increasing posture problems. Along with backache, this can cause dexterity impairment as well as loss of agility, coordination, and balance.

We've already established that hormonal changes affect your ligaments. What we haven't mentioned is that this too can lead to injury, especially as joints in the spine become less stable to accommodate your growing baby.

SHE WORKS HARD FOR HER MONEY

I had a longtime patient I'll call Anne. She was overjoyed when she learned that she was pregnant, but we both knew it was not going to be an easy nine months. First of all, Anne had previously suffered a disc herniation that had required surgical intervention. Second, she has type 2 diabetes. And to further complicate the situation, she worked a full-time job that she would not be leaving until right before delivery.

As soon as I learned she was pregnant, I started monitoring her condition closely as did her medical doctor because of the diabetes and lower-back issues.

Anne's job required her to sit most of the day, which sounds like the perfect job for an expectant mom. It isn't. Sitting for extended periods of time causes severe compression of the spine, with the possibility of disc disruption. Since she had already suffered a herniated disc, she was at risk of experiencing another disc injury to her surgically repaired spinal column.

Anne was working eight to ten hours a day and soon began showing signs of exhaustion. She was getting limited sleep and getting limited exercise because of her fatigue level.

By the time she was in her third trimester, her ankles were so swollen that they left rings where her socks rode on her legs. It was apparent that her sitting all day with the weight of the baby compressing the larger blood vessels of the pelvis and thighs was preventing good venous return of blood to the heart, causing this terrible edema around her ankles.

The solution was massage. The massage therapist in our office worked hard to get Anne's blood flow stimulated in her extremities whenever she could get into the office.

Everyone in my office appreciated the fact that Anne was working hard at her job and at bringing a new life into this world. Today, mother and daughter are doing great.

Reach distance.

You don't need to be reminded that as your pregnancy progresses, your abdomen grows. That means you need to lift and maneuver objects farther away from your body than you did just a few months ago. If you've always had a comfortable reach of fifteen inches, you'll now probably need to reach twenty inches to accomplish the exact same task.

No, your arms didn't shrink. Now you just have a bundle of joy between where you are and whatever it is you're reaching for.

In order to compensate, you put additional strain on your arms, shoulders, and lower back. You may even twist your back so you can reach sideways to extend your arm. The result is that you are no longer lifting the object squarely, and you may be lifting something with one hand that you would normally lift with two.

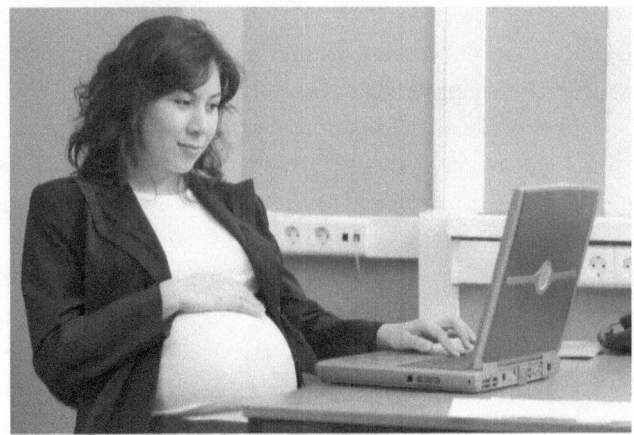

If you repeat that reaching motion multiple times throughout the day, day after day, back pain is inevitable.

Not to get overly technical, but bear with me for a moment. If you normally lift a ten-pound object, your body is absorbing sixty-five pounds of pressure on your lower back. In your third trimester, because you now need to lift and maneuver the same ten-pound object farther away from your body, you're increasing the load on your spine to about 150 pounds of pressure—an increase of 230 percent!

Ouch. My back hurts just thinking about it.

Unfortunately, few (if any) *anthropometric* (big word speaks of human body measurement) studies of pregnant women have been conducted. I've never seen one, and believe me, I've looked. So it is difficult to find standardized information on appropriate workstation design. My recommendation is to understand the potential pitfalls of your work site and to consider things like working surface height and the positioning of any repetitive tasks in relation to your reach. To avoid stretching, you'll probably need to move some things around as your pregnancy progresses, but it will pay off in the end when you minimize or, hopefully, eliminate back pain and long-term back problems.

Balance.

You already know that your continually shifting center of gravity negatively impacts your balance. Your ever-changing weight has a similar effect. Before you became pregnant, your center of gravity was located in front of your spine, level with your kidneys. As your growing baby shifts your center of gravity forward, balance becomes an issue.

You'll also find that your pregnancy makes you more awkward and easily fatigued. Coupled with your questionable balance, any job that requires quick reaction time or work on elevated surfaces becomes more dangerous. Work on platforms or even the use of step stools present a hazard for working moms-to-be.

My experience is that most responsible, caring employers and certainly most coworkers understand that your pregnancy requires that you stand with your feet planted firmly on the ground. My recommendation is that you stay on this side of dumb and don't insist that you can do it, whatever *it* is. Your baby, your back, and your well-being require that you modify what you ask your body to endure while you're pregnant.

Let Mary Jo climb the ladder for you when you're pregnant. Just remember to do the same thing for her when your conditions are reversed.

Lifting.

This is the biggest concern I have because when you bend to lift an object, you're not only elevating the weight of the object, you're also raising the additional weight of the baby. And you're doing it with muscles and ligaments that are already being loosened and stressed beyond normal levels.

Pelvic muscles relax, and spine joints become less stable, both of which increase the risk of back injury.

Nobody wants to be considered weak. It's a cultural embarrassment. Get over it. Obviously, pregnancy changes the amount of weight you can lift safely. According to a study conducted by the University of Texas that compared upper-limb strength of pregnant and nonpregnant women in the workplace, it was found that, not surprisingly, nonpregnant women were *significantly* stronger. The researchers concluded that this finding had safety implications for both the mother and the fetus. They recommended that lifting criteria be taken into consideration when assigning job tasks.

The American Medical Women's Association recommends that risk management programs include a weight restriction of twenty-five pounds for pregnant women.

My clinical experience disagrees with that distinguished body of ten thousand female doctors. I'd reduce the high end of lifting 20 percent. I firmly believe that anything over twenty pounds puts your back at risk.

If potentially damaging your back weren't enough, here are some other very real ways lifting can negatively impact your pregnancy and your baby:

Those of you considering pumping iron, please take note of the following:

♦ Muscular activity alters blood flow in the body, decreasing blood flow to the uterus, and placenta frequently resulting in low birth weight.

♦ Heavy lifting has been shown to affect intraabdominal pressures that may provoke uterine contractions.

♦ In early pregnancy, heavy lifting in conjunction with physical effort like bending movements has been associated with an increase in spontaneous abortion—miscarriage.

♦ Significant physical exertion may lead to hormone disturbances, hyperthermia, and nutritional deficits.

Standing.

Although it sounds nonthreatening enough, standing for extended periods of time can also cause back problems when you're pregnant.

As your pregnancy progresses into the later stages, the curve of your lower back increases, which means your back muscles need to work harder to help you maintain your balance and upright position. The result is often pain in your lower back.

Not related to your back but of concern for your pregnancy is a study by the Association of Women's Health, Obstetric and Neonatal Nurses that found that women who stand more than four to six hours a day had an increased rate of preterm deliveries.

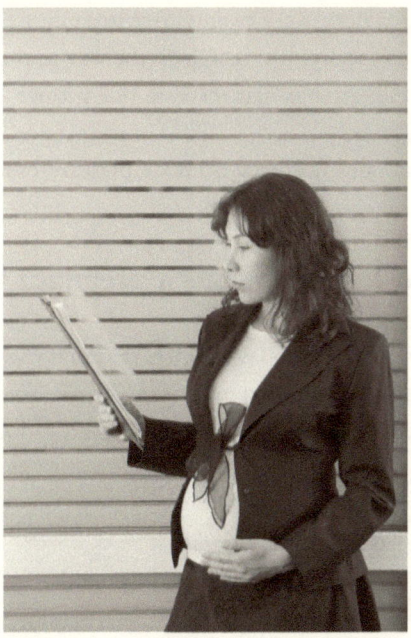

Sitting.

Many working expectant mothers read about a job where you sit all day and ask, "Where do I sign up?" What, they wonder, is the downside?

Whether you are pregnant or not, sitting for an extended period of time, more than two hours, creates a constant load on the intervertebral discs of the spine. This pressure causes loss of fluid in the disc, reducing its thickness. This loss of disc height can cause excess stress on the bony joints and leave you susceptible to disc herniation.

When you add pregnancy to the back challenges associated with a desk job, you significantly complicate the situation. Especially in your second and third trimesters, sitting can cause compression of your deep pelvic blood vessels, which results in swelling over your ankles and feet.

For disc compression caused by sitting for long periods of time, the best thing you can do to relieve the pressure is to lie down for one hour for every hour you sit. As soon as you get home from work, lie down for an hour. "What about dinner?" you worry. Buy a copy of Rachael Ray's *30 Minute Meals*. Then point the man in your life toward the kitchen. Lie down while he cooks dinner. (If he doesn't embrace the idea, let him read this book so he knows it's *doctor's orders*.) That hour of resting your back, coupled with a good night's sleep, should counteract the damage done by sitting.

For the pregnancy complications of sitting, there are several things you should do to reduce swelling of your feet and ankles as well as lower back fatigue:

♦ Get up from your desk every twenty to thirty minutes.
♦ Use a chair that supports your thigh all the way to the knee.
♦ Make sure the chair has armrests at the proper height to reduce neck stressors.
♦ Get a foot stool, and use it to decrease pressure over the deep pelvic blood vessels.

How can I still work as a pregnant woman?

I realize that the reality of life today requires that many women continue working through their pregnancy. What you need to do is modify your work life. If your employer doesn't embrace these recommendations, just tell them it's "doctor's orders."

Modifications:

♦ Ask to be assigned less physical tasks.
♦ Restrict lifting to no more than twenty pounds, and stop lifting altogether during the third trimester.

- Adjust work hours—for example, flexible scheduling, day shift instead of night, etc.
- Vary tasks to avoid static posture for long periods of time.
- Install footrests, whether you are seated or standing, so that one foot can be alternately raised.
- Limit standing time to less than three hours a day.
- Be aware that the firm edge of your chair or stool can obstruct blood vessels in your legs, which can ultimately result in blood clots.
- Modify your break schedule, for example, shorter more frequent breaks.
- Eliminate working at heights, such as ladders or step stools.
- Walking in moderation is encouraged throughout your pregnancy. Walking causes the leg veins to pump blood upward from the feet and helps prevent minor swelling of the ankles.

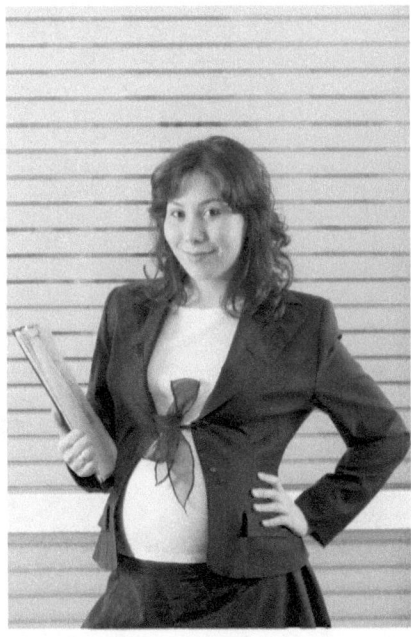

SECTION 3

YOUR BABY'S BIG DAY

CHAPTER 11

YOUR LABOR AND DELIVERY

How will all of this work on my back help during childbirth?

Once that small miracle of life in your belly decides to make his or her debut, it's easy to start forgetting about the role your back plays in the whole process. That's why I'm going to take this chapter to discuss the mechanics behind the pelvis and birth canal and what you have worked so hard for during this pregnancy.

Even if the care and feeding of your spine for nine months may not have seemed critical previously, it's during the delivery when you may see the greatest benefit.

It has been my experience that women who have diligently done the mechanical work on their pelvis and spine throughout their pregnancy experience shorter deliveries and actual push time.

I'm not suggesting that labor and delivery won't be any more inconvenient than having your hair done. I'm just observing that no matter how hard it is, it would be a whole lot harder if you hadn't done the preparation work.

THE IMPATIENT PATIENT

I am the chiropractor for the Colorado Eagles professional ice hockey team. We do our best to keep a healthy team on the ice. One of the player's wives, whom I'll call Lisa, came into the office one afternoon and announced that she was ready to have her second baby.

She was very pregnant, about thirty-nine weeks. Lisa was very nice about everything, but she was adamant that she wanted to be done with the pregnancy.

As a hockey wife, she characterized her feelings by saying, "The third period's over. We're waiting for the buzzer to end the game."

Lisa reported that she had little to no pain over her lower back and no neck discomfort. I could empathize with Lisa because with our fourth child, Gina had hit a similar wall.

I examined Lisa and determined that she was in good physical condition. I made sure her pelvis was properly aligned and ready to have the baby.

She made a follow-up appointment that we both hoped she'd miss because she would have had the baby in the interim.

It didn't happen. She showed up for the appointment, and I turned to acupuncture.

Many medical practitioners look at stimulating childbirth as some kind of heresy. (These are the same guys who pull out their calendars and schedule a C-section.)

The body is an amazing organism that knows precisely what to do when given the proper information. Lisa's ob-gyn was in favor of my doing anything I could to help her along.

Lisa was a trooper. I did a very small acupuncture pattern, and we were both very optimistic when she left although she did make an appointment for later in the week.

She showed up for the third appointment and was worried that her hockey player husband would be out of town on a road trip with the team and would miss the birth.

This time, we pulled out all of the stops using acupuncture and electric stimulation over the birth stimulation points. Lisa experienced movement of the baby.

A few weeks later, Lisa, her husband, and the new baby came into the office. She told me that she had started contractions and was in the hospital within two hours after our last treatment.

Third-period buzzer. Game over. Home team wins!

What do I need to know about my pelvis?

You're probably sitting there holding this book and thinking to yourself, "My pelvis is nothing more than a bony structure. What's the big deal?"

The big deal is the fact that your baby is going to pass through that bone and that your body is going to have to accommodate that short journey.

What you need to know about your pelvis isn't the bone—it's the ligaments surrounding it. Ligaments hold bony structures together; and as we discussed in an earlier chapter, the hormones naturally produced during pregnancy loosen ligaments, especially the ligaments of your pelvis.

And there are *lots* of ligaments lining your pelvis, too many to bore you with by listing them here. The thing you need to know is that the ligaments are instrumental in the mechanical process of delivery.

The ligaments within and around your pelvis are among the strongest in your body because they function as the anchor for the trunk of your body. Whenever you stand up, those are the ligaments that bear the brunt of your resting tension weight.

Are you going to tell me more about my pelvis than I want to know?

I probably already did. There is greater detail at the end of this book in appendix C, *The Anatomy of Your Pelvis*. It discusses the structure—the bones that comprise your pelvis, as well as the connecting ligaments. It goes on to give you some information about hormones. I tried to give you the knowledge you need to understand what's happening to your body through your labor process.

Early-stage labor

In the early stage of labor, the hip flexor muscles are stretched, causing the pelvis to tip forward and the apex (tip) of the sacrum to move forward as well. This is to allow for the pelvic brim to open, allowing the baby to descend lower in the pelvis.

Late-stage labor

Flexion of your hips with your knees bent for the pushing stage tends to tilt the pelvis back, causing a decrease in the diameter of the pelvic brim but opening the pelvic outlet. This is the expulsive stage of labor. It allows the baby's head to move past the pelvic outlet.

The difference from flexion to extension of the sacrum is measured in millimeters.

What happens if my pelvis is misaligned?

Misalignments of the pelvis for whatever reason can have serious consequences during labor. Having your pelvic alignment off by as little as five millimeters (about a fifth of an inch) can be the difference between an open pelvic outlet and a condition that obstructs the baby's descent.

Not all birthing problems can be avoided with mechanical intervention, of course. But pelvic misalignment is one condition that can be corrected prior to labor.

The chiropractor on your health care team is the person to go to for pelvic alignment. He or she will examine you and correct any issues to make sure that the pelvic brim and outlet are aligned properly. It is especially important that you attend all of your appointments with your chiropractor in the last few weeks before you are scheduled to deliver.

CHAPTER 12

LABOR AND NECK PAIN AND HEADACHES

Why am I worried about my neck and my head?

I'm in the middle of giving birth here!

When you're in active labor, the last thing you're worrying about is the headache you're going to have next week. But the reality of the situation is that there is a great deal of potential for damage to your neck during the late stages of labor. Neck (or cervical spine) injury is a common cause for severe headaches that may last for months after you've given birth.

Here's what happens:

> During the stage when you're being told to push, most women lift their heads from the bed and strain with everything they've got. Their neck muscles tense, and blood vessels are visible through their skin. Their beet-red faces grimace with herculean effort.

Your "coach" . . . may help you push the baby out of your womb by pushing on the back of your neck like it's a stubborn lawn chair.

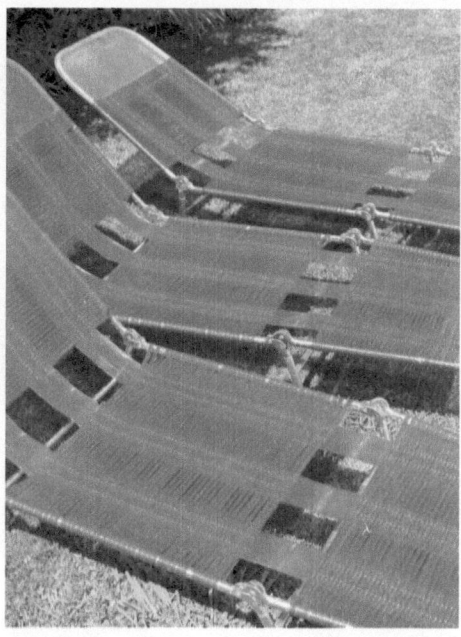

In many cases, your "coach," ever helpful chap that he is, may help you push the baby out of your womb by pushing on the back of your neck like it's a stubborn lawn chair. Sure, he knows intellectually that there's no way to move the baby in your belly by using all of his strength to ram your chin into your chest; but if you're straining in that position, he wants to fix your problem for you. It's something we guys do, regardless of how moronic it sounds in more sober moments.

All of this bearing down causes undue pressure on your neck. And yes, injury can occur to joints, muscles, ligaments, and even cervical vertebrae.

Frankly, shoving your head to your chest, with or without "help," is probably the worst possible position for your neck while bearing down for an hour or more. You can cause trauma to the intervertebral discs in your neck. I've also seen cases where moms have caused damage to their lower back as well.

Frankly, shoving your head to your chest . . . is probably the worst possible position for your neck.

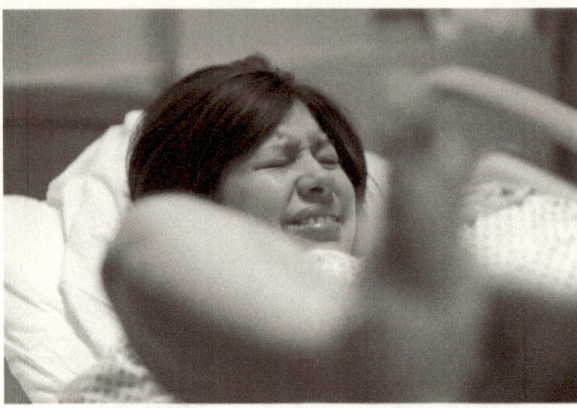

At the very least, you can *strain a muscle*, which means the muscle fibers pull and tear. The end result is the neck tension of labor can cause bony alignment issues, resulting in neck pain and headaches for months after the birth. You probably won't attribute the discomfort to the blessed event because your attention during labor is usually focused on another area of your anatomy.

During labor, you need to consciously keep your head flat or, at least, in a straight line on the bed and resist the natural urge to lift your head. Make sure your coach knows how much his helping could hurt long term. Instead of grappling with your back, he needs to quietly remind you to resist clamping your chin to your chest.

It would also be wise to tell your coach ahead of time that he needs to leave the pushing to the expert—you.

CHAPTER 13

THE OTHER SIDE OF LABOR PAINS

How does my back impact childbirth?

When most women think about *labor pains*, they are referring to the discomfort they experience within the uterus that accompanies contractions. There are many other areas where you may feel pain during labor, though. Often, pain will occur in areas where the ligaments that hold the uterus in place are stressed. Occasionally, there will be pain at the joints, especially the pubic symphysis and the sacroiliac joints. Sometimes, the cervix opening and stretching is painful. A few women experience pain in their thighs as the baby is moving down the birth canal.

About one in four women (25 percent) are faced with labor pains on the posterior side of their bodies: the dreaded *back labor*. While pain in the back is not uncommon during contractions, it is the pain that lingers after the contraction is gone that defines true back labor.

Okay, you're thinking, "Back labor doesn't sound like something I want. How do I prevent it?"

What is back labor?

Back labor is most often caused by the position of the baby's head, usually in the *occiput posterior* position, frequently shortened simply to *OP*. This is when your baby is in the head-down position in your uterus but with his or her nose facing your abdomen.

This leaves the hardest part of the baby, the back of the skull, resting on the bony part of your spine, your sacrum.

Back labor is most often caused by the position of the baby's head.

The front or *anterior* of the sacrum (the part that is facing your baby) is where some of the nerve roots exit your spinal cord. When the back of the baby's head (the occiput) rubs up against the sacrum, you experience pain over the top of the sacrum. Voila, back labor.

How can I prevent back labor?

Okay, here's the bad news: You can't prevent back labor. Because it is caused by the position the baby takes when the little darling finally decides to make his or her grand entrance, there is no preparation or accommodation you can make beforehand.

Face it, this may be the first time your offspring puts you in an uncomfortable position; but judging from my four kids, it won't be the last.

How can I cope with back labor?

That's a better question. There are actually some fairly simple things you can do to deal with the pain of back labor.

1. **Get the baby to change positions.**
   I suggested jumping jacks to my wife. She hit me. Hard. Your ob-gyn or midwife may have a better idea to help get the baby to spin 180 degrees.
2. **Take some steps to relieve the pain.**

   a. **Take advantage of gravity.** The simplest thing is to get up on all fours. Sure, it's not a traditional birthing position; but gravity will drop the baby away from your spine, relieving the pressure. When you're on your hands and knees, the baby is tipped slightly out of the pelvis, giving it more room to rotate. Due to the decreased pressure on the cervix, many moms experience less pain during the contractions. This position is also terrific for your coach to apply counterpressure to your lower back.

b.   **Do *pelvic tilts*.** (See chapter 7 with stretches.)

Pelvic tilts are a common abdominal exercise done on your hands and knees as if you were going to crawl. Your arms should be fully extended and straight so that the floor, your legs, your back, and your arms form the four sides of a square. You start with your back straight (not arched up or down) with your stomach pulled up. Next, slowly relax your lower back, and allow your pelvis to tilt forward comfortably. Hold this position for a couple of seconds, and then pull your back and pelvis into the straight (less-relaxed) position. This cycle should be repeated slowly in a regular motion. Try to do this exercise using the muscles in the lower part of your body.

3.   **Use counterpressure.**

Have your coach use his hands and push your lower back between contractions, usually at or just above the sacrum. This will help counter the pressure where you are feeling the most pain.

PERSONAL ~~EXPERIENCE~~ OBSERVATION

Okay, it didn't happen to me, but I was there. My wife had back labor with Lauren, our first child. During the later stages of her labor, Gina informed me and her delivery team through frank verbal communication at a notably higher-than-normal volume that she was experiencing extreme pain over the top of her sacrum.

Typing the word PAIN#%&@!!! in capital letters and putting it in boldface doesn't really give you a clear understanding of the intensity of the discomfort Gina experienced.

To help relieve her pain, I used the counterpressure method described here by using my thumbs over the top of her sacrum. I pushed as hard as I could, and when my thumbs would wear out, our massage therapist took over. I know what you moms are thinking, "Boohoo, poor guy went through labor and got tired thumbs." I know I felt terrible about feeling sorry for myself at the time. I remember thinking how her back must have felt!

4.   **Apply hot or cold.**

Sometimes, it's helpful to take a warm bath or aim a water shower at your lower back. You could also use something like a warm pad or a cold pack or a warmed or cooled wet towel. How can you tell whether you need heat or coolness? In my clinical experience, there's no rule of thumb. Try them both. The one that works for you is the right answer.

5. **Make use of back rubs.**

   Having your coach give you a back rub on your lower back, especially using a tennis ball or other round objects, can oftentimes help relieve discomfort. (And it'll save your coach's fingers and thumbs.)

6. **Employ essential oils.**

   Just like rubbing BENGAY or Icy Hot on a muscle pain, some essential oils can reduce pain naturally. You may want to try proven pain-relieving oils like eucalyptus, peppermint, lavender, or sage.

7. **Accept an epidural or spinal anesthesia.**

   This is the least attractive alternative, both from the perspective of the baby's birth and from your long-term medical standpoint. However, there are times when there is no other solution. If you absolutely need it, take the shot. You won't feel back pain. You also won't feel your thighs—or even your feet.

Epidural side effects.

Having never given birth, I'm not in a position to discourage anyone from using whatever means available to alleviate pain and suffering. However, I know about some potential side effects to spinal anesthesia that you should discuss with your ob-gyn or midwife prior to your due date.

Short-term concerns for moms:

 ◆ dural puncture*
 ◆ low blood pressure
 ◆ nausea, vomiting, shivering
 ◆ prolonged labor
 ◆ toxic drug reactions
 ◆ convulsions
 ◆ headache (slight to severe)
 ◆ septic meningitis
 ◆ allergic shock
 ◆ cardiac arrest
 ◆ respiratory insufficiency
 ◆ feelings of emotional detachment

---

* **Dural puncture.** The dura is the outermost fibrous membrane that covers the spinal cord. Accidental puncture during administration of an epidural anesthetic can lead to complications like headache, backache, nerve damage, and even brain damage.

Long-term concerns for moms:

- neurological complications
- backache (weeks to years)
- postpartum feelings of regret
- fecal and urinary incontinence
- bladder dysfunction
- loss of perineal sensation
- loss of sexual function
- paresthesia ("pins and needles")

Health concerns for the baby:

- direct drug toxicity
- drowsiness at birth
- poor-sucking reflex
- neonatal jaundice
- fetal distress—abnormal fetal heart rate (FHR)
- poor muscle strength in first hours
- decreased maternal-infant bonding

EPIDURAL BLOOD PATCH

While we just listed potential side effects of the epidural that you need to be aware of, I'm not totally against them. They are one of the tools available to your health care team and should be used when appropriate. As I alluded to in the preface of this book, if mankind depended on men to bear children, our species would have become extinct long ago.

The team approach can help even after you've delivered your baby. The case of Barb comes to mind.

Barb went through pregnancy with your usual uncomfortable periods related to her lower back, which we relieved as needed. She rarely had trouble with either neck or upper-back pain.

Throughout her pregnancy, Barb was great about drinking water and watching sodium intake.

She went into labor, and everything went okay with the birth.

After giving birth, though, she began suffering extreme headaches. Pounding pain in her head brought her to my office for relief.

Knowing Barb's history, I found it strange for her to be having such bad headaches, but I wasn't overly concerned. As we learned in the birthing section of this book, postpartum headaches can sometimes be brought on by the trauma of the birth itself.

I learned that Barb had neck stiffness but no numbness or radiating tingling into her upper extremities. She explained that she had done as I had instructed and kept her head out of flexion as much as she could during her labor and delivery.

She explained that she did have an epidural.

At that point, we were five days postpartum. I checked her spine to find very rigid muscles, but her alignment was not bad at all.

Seeing nothing mechanical that would cause her headaches, I became concerned about a possible cerebral spinal fluid leak at the epidural injection site on her spinal cord. Headaches are fairly common with an epidural, but they usually resolve within a day or two. Five days was too long for a typical epidural headache.

We called Barb's obstetrician from our office, and they told her to come right over. What they discovered was a tear in the dura (the sack around the spinal cord) where she received her epidural injection. With a procedure called a blood patch, the anesthesiologist was able to fix her problem. Within a week, she was doing great and enjoying life and her baby headache free.

Without a single spinal correction in my office, I was able to help Barb resolve her headaches.

This was a great example of how members of Barb's health care team worked together for the common good of the patient.

SECTION 4

AFTER YOU'VE GIVEN BIRTH

CHAPTER 14

YOUR BACK PAIN (PART 2)

How can I avoid hurting my back after I've given birth?

After you get home from the hospital, your back has a host of new issues to confront, many of which can cause back pain and even long-term back damage if not properly managed. As unfair as it sounds, you can do everything right for your back during your pregnancy, have a short push-time birth, and still end up with a nagging backache months or even years later.

How?

You'll be doing things with your body that are out of the ordinary—bathing someone else, nursing, pushing a stroller, loading a car seat, and changing diapers, for example.

DON'T THROW YOUR BACK OUT WITH YOUR BABY'S BATHWATER

I have to admit, I didn't really understand the dynamics of your back and your baby's bath time until Gina and I had kids of our own. To put it bluntly, your lower back is at great risk of injury when you're bathing your baby.

Many years ago, before I was a dad, I had a patient I'll call Claire. Claire was a diligent patient throughout her pregnancy. She followed doctor's orders to the letter and did very well. She had a good birth and was checked out postpartum a few weeks after the birth, and everything was going great.

Then one day, Claire came into the office without an appointment. She was suffering from severe low-back pain. We went through her history, and she explained that she was giving the baby a bath in the sink. Claire's baby, Sara, was an adorable little girl who weighed over eight pounds at birth.

It seems Claire was bathing Sara in a dandy invention called a baby bathing hammock. I asked her about positioning and learned that Claire was standing in slight rotation and bent slightly at the waist pressed up against the countertop. In other words, she had to twist her body to bathe the baby.

That led to my next question, "How long do you typically stand in that position."

"Ten to fifteen minutes," Claire answered. "I know it doesn't take that long to wash her little body, but she loves playing in the bathwater, and it's a great bonding time for us."

Indeed, bath time is a wonderful experience for the parent and the baby.

The problem came to a head one evening when Claire's back started to tighten up. As she retold the story, I understood how terrified she was that she might drop her baby when she felt a sharp stabbing pain in her back.

Claire had suffered a small annular tear of one of her lumbar discs due to many complicating factors, one of which was the delivery itself. Another contributing issue, though, was her back-stressing position while bathing little Sara nightly in the sink.

We treated Claire, and she was roughly 50 percent better after the first treatment. Four adjustments and a week and a half later, you would have never guessed she had anything wrong with her back at all.

Rick, Claire's husband, brought her to her appointments; and I recruited him to help with bath time. Frankly, your risk of injury is greatly reduced if you use the team approach whenever possible, especially in the first four weeks postpartum.

How can bathing my eight-pound baby hurt my back?

First of all, the baby isn't going to stay eight pounds for very long. And second, how many times have you bent over anything for a long period of time every day and not felt a little stiffness in your back? Add to that your loosened ligaments and a prolonged awkward position that includes lifting a wiggling, slippery eight-pound weight and you'll start to see what I'm getting at here.

Bath time is a great time of the day for both you and your baby. Speaking from experience, dads enjoy the time too. I genuinely have fun bathing my kids, especially when they're very little.

But baby baths can lead to bad backs.

Baby baths can lead to bad backs.

Sponge baths.

Initially, as a new parent, I recommend sponge baths. Let's face it, the little rascal isn't out running in the yard getting grimy and sweaty. He or she isn't going to get *that* dirty. With a sponge bath, you have control over the height of the washing surface, and you can minimize bending and lifting. You also don't need to continually support your baby's head in the water, so you have two hands free.

I recommend sponge baths initially for the first three to four weeks because they'll allow your body, and especially your back, to recover from labor and delivery.

Sink baths.

Eventually, you'll graduate to the sink or possibly a small bathing tub sitting on a counter. Sinks or small portable tubs have advantages because you can remain standing. The challenge to your back comes from the continual slight flexion and rotation that you'll be required to perform. In many instances, I have seen mothers who aren't able to stand square to the sink because of the size of the sink or tub or because of the demands for washing the baby's hair.

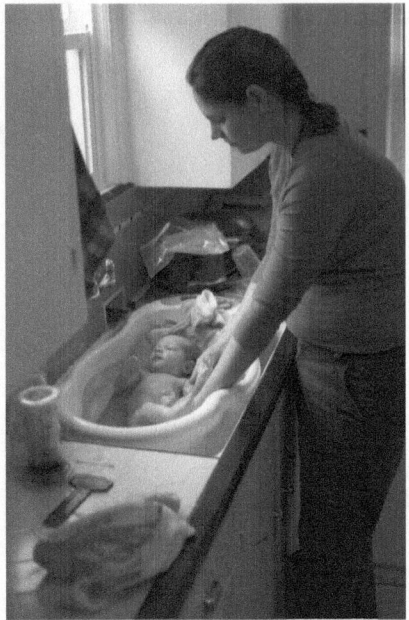

Many mothers who have recently gone through labor and delivery can be susceptible to back strain in this position, placing stress on the lumbar discs.

Standing at the sink or counter can often be tolerated until the moment when the bath ends and the drying begins. As you start to lift this eight-, ten-, or twelve-pound precious little slippery person out of the sink, you load your spine because, of course, you lifted by straightening your slightly bent back.

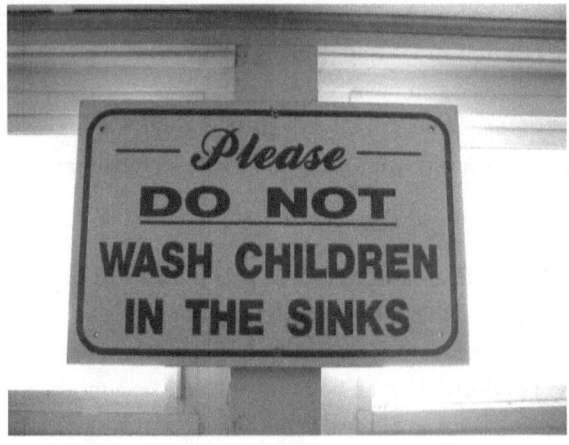

Whoa! Little herky-jerky baby. And ouch!

Before you know it, you have a tight and painful lower back.

Bathtub baths.

Eventually, as your baby gets bigger, you'll move to the bathtub at bath time. By then, your baby has doubled or tripled his or her birth weight. You're lifting more than twenty pounds over a nineteen-inch barrier and bending over to support that weight for the duration of the bath.

The stress on your back from bending at your waist (flexion) is tremendous; and by kneeling, bending, and extending over the tub, you place tremendous shearing force throughout your lower back. You can easily cause back problems for years to come.

When you think about it, it would be better for your back if the kid stayed dirty for the first couple of years.

Recommended bathing technique.

The best way to bathe your baby is to get into the tub with him or her. You won't be forced to bend for an extended period of time, and you will have greater control of your baby in the water.

The best way to bathe your baby is to get into the tub with him or her.

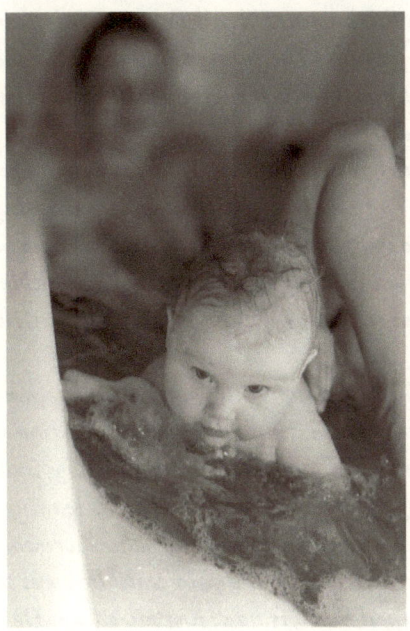

From my experience, this is a great time for everyone involved. You get to play with your baby, and your baby gets to play with you. Talk about quality time and getting to know each other!

As far as getting your baby out of the tub, I suggest that whichever parent isn't in the tub should be nearby so the baby can be handed out with neither parent experiencing back strain.

TUBBY DADDY

Here's some comic relief for everyone but the poor guy who walked into my office with postpartum back pain. That's right, I said guy.

First, you have to understand a strange medical phenomenon that they don't teach us doctors, but that I have observed many, many times in my practice: A great many men gain weight when their wives are pregnant. Go figure. There is no medical or even logical explanation for this, and to my knowledge, nobody has ever done a study about the condition.

I have to admit it: I'm one of those guys. I gained weight with each of my children. For me, it was as though Gina was secreting a pheromone that caused me to eat chocolate. (If she's going to blame me for getting her pregnant, it's only fair that I blame her for my excess poundage. Right? Ladies . . . ?)

Okay, well, I've got this patient I'll call Tubby. While Tubby's wife was pregnant, he put on fifteen extra pounds. The funny thing was that she looked great while he had to go out and buy pants with a bigger waist size. (Here's an idea, maternity pants for expectant dads.)

Just like an expectant or new mother, Tubby's center of gravity changed, just not as quickly as his wife's. The extra weight, though, was stressing the joints and discs in his lower back trying to support his new belly and his new baby-related activities.

When Tubby hobbled into my office, he was barely able to walk. This guy was limping like he invented it. Tubby was an established patient, but I had never seen him in this bad shape.

"Tub," I said, "What'd you do? Quit your job and become a professional hot dog eater?" Tubby glared at me and didn't dignify the question with an answer.

I got down to business and took a new health history, and that's when he told me the story. He was giving his new son a bath. He was leaning all his newly acquired weight on the lip of a nineteen-inch bathtub while scrubbing his brand-new son. He was having fun interacting with the baby until he went to get the giggling fellow from the tub. He explained how his back just seized up. He couldn't move!

Fortunately, his wife was home and was able to take care of the little guy. The big guy was another story.

It took great effort for Tubby to get into my office. It took him four treatments to get everything back into place and functioning properly. Needless to say, he learned his lesson and started following my bathing recommendations, just as his healthy, happy wife had been doing all along.

How can carrying my kids on my hip hurt my back?

Frequently, new mothers come to my clinic with lower-back pain that has more to do with the new baby's siblings than with the new baby. We've all seen it: moms carrying two—and three-year-old kids on their hips (the top of your ilium). Note: Children cannot ride on a guy's hips because our love handles get in the way.

Before I had children, it was easy to pronounce my naïve instruction to mothers: "Don't carry your children on your hips."

Like that was ever going to happen.

As much as the doctor side of me wants to stop you from carrying your kids on your hips, the dad side of me realizes that it is totally natural way for you to carry your babies and young children.

If this is your first baby, your back will slowly regain strength; so as your bundle of joy gets heavier, you'll be able to accommodate the weight. I would urge you to shift sides frequently so neither hip is stressed.

The more serious back pain problems come from carrying your baby's siblings shortly after you've given birth. Your ligaments have not had time to tighten, and the twenty or more pounds of big brother or sister puts undue stress on your back. Back pain is likely to follow.

Still, you have a little pair of arms reaching up to you and shouting, "Up, up, up!" The doctor side of me says, "So?"

The dad side of me knows that you have a little guilt thing going on about not giving your older children the attention they have come to expect. You don't want them to resent the new baby. You love them just as much.

One idea is to sit your older children down and explain to them some of the physiological changes your body has gone through giving birth to their new brother or sister. Remind them that it only *seems* like you are giving all your love to the new baby. They should react with the same understanding and compassion the baby's dad exhibits when you explain the same things to him.

Hey, it was an idea. I never said it was a good idea.

A more realistic approach would be to hold your older children on your lap, sitting on a chair when the baby is down for a nap or otherwise occupied. When you absolutely have to pick them up, change sides frequently, and put them down as quickly as possible.

Your new baby needs to be held and touched, but so do your other kids.

I recommend that you try to wean your older children from being carried to minimize damage to your back.

Whenever possible, let the dad do the heavy lifting. When he is available, put him in charge of carrying all siblings, backpacks, toys, and diaper bags. Not only will this save on wear and tear of the mom's back, but it is a great way for the dad to build relationships with his children. Carrying little kids on your shoulders goes a long way in convincing them that you are the strongest daddy on earth.

How can loading my baby into a car seat hurt my back?

At my chiropractic practice, we know for a fact that car seats are great for our business because, unfortunately, they are terrible for your back.

First of all, many parents carry their newborn in their car seat. Handy, right? Wait until you wrestle with one of the crazy crooked handle models. But regardless of the handle design, I have yet to encounter a car seat that gives you equal weight distribution.

My recommendation would be to look for a light but sturdy car seat with a good safety rating and record. Here in the United States, the National Highway Traffic Safety Administration (NHTSA) rates car seats by brand name and model. Consumers Union, publisher of *Consumer Reports* magazine, has also rated car seats in the past.

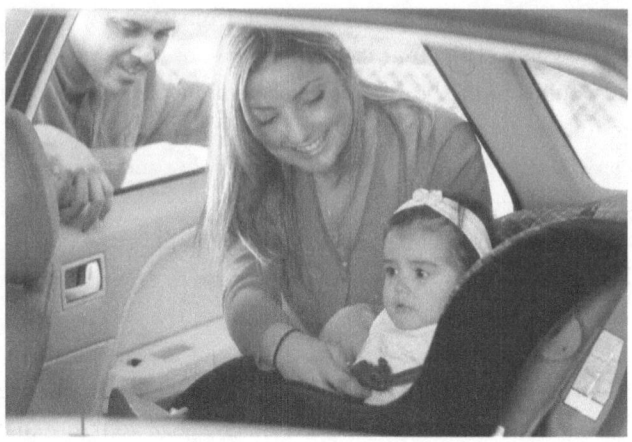

Carrying an ever-growing baby awkwardly in front of you can't help but cause compression and torsion of your spine, particularly your lower back. And I have seen many car seat models that are ridiculously heavy.

Carrying an ever-growing baby awkwardly in front of you can't help but cause compression and torsion of your spine.

When you transport the baby in the car seat, carry it with your hands together and very close to the center of your torso, just below your breastbone.

Whenever possible, push your baby in a stroller. As you gain experience in your baby education, you'll realize that a small sturdy stroller is an invaluable aid. In fact, by the time we had our third child, I was surprised whenever I saw my wife carry our baby in the car seat. She'd leave the car seat in the car (imagine that!). By our fourth child, we got really smart and discovered a car seat that just hooks into the stroller.

THE LATEST DESIGN DOESN'T ALWAYS MEAN GOOD

I'm frequently reminded that the people who design baby equipment are usually men. There's no other explanation for how some products can be so trendy "cool," but potentially harmful to a woman recovering from giving birth.

There's a misconception that the more state-of-the-art the car seat or stroller, the better you are as a parent. I think baby goods salespeople start salivating the moment they hear that their customer is a first-time parent. Remember, your

THE OTHER SIDE OF PREGNANCY

parents probably pushed you around in a ten-dollar umbrella stroller, and you turned out just fine. Make sure the equipment you buy is good for your baby and good for you. It's no fun being the coolest mom on the block if you're in constant pain.

I have a longtime patient whom I'll call Lynn. She was a first-time mother of a happy and healthy young man named Jayden. Before her delivery, Lynn and I had agreed that she'd come in for a check-up shortly after she was settled back home with her new baby.

By the time she was settled enough to make an appointment with my office, Jayden was a little over six months old, roughly a half year overdue.

I didn't take it personally. I know from experience that a new mom's life is no longer her own. The baby monopolizes your time. And you are often so sleep deprived that when you get a few moments to yourself, you'd rather take a nap than visit your faithful old chiropractor.

Waiting in the hallway as my assistant led Lynn to the treatment room, I was dismayed to see that Lynn had her hips stuck out one way, and her arm stuck out the other as she carried a state-of-the-art crooked handle car seat. Her pelvis, back, shoulder, elbow, and wrist were all being stressed by carrying the weight of the baby-filled car seat out to the side of her body. Figure about ten pounds for the car seat and twenty pounds for the baby and she's walking along trying to balance about thirty pounds off to the side of her hips.

She looked more contorted than cool.

I also noticed that her bundle of joy was truly a bundle. Little Jayden was wrapped in a blanket so tightly, he reminded me of a burrito. I was amazed that she had been able to even buckle him into the seat. As I watched Lynn approach, I saw that the baby was bouncing back and forth like a rolling ship in a storm. It was obvious to me that the baby had been encased in the blanket for his own protection.

I didn't need too much time to diagnose her issues. She had neck muscle strain with the signs of the early stages of shoulder tendonitis. Her lower-back pain came from strain and stress with pelvic misalignment.

I asked about postpartum massage work and was disappointed but not surprised when her response was, "No, I haven't gotten around to it." Because it was obvious to both of us, I resisted the urge to lecture her that she was paying me good money and then not taking my advice to get out of this pain.

I corrected her pelvis and spine and treated her shoulder with therapeutic ultrasound. I also gave her strong encouragement to get a couple massages over the next few weeks. I also recommended that she use her stroller as much as possible when moving Jayden from point A to point B.

She promised to use the stroller and get the massages then bent down to pick up her car seat from Hades. I had patients in the waiting room, but I really didn't want to see my work wrecked before she even pulled out of our parking lot. So I volunteered to carry Jayden to her car.

She was actually relieved and readily agreed. I understood more fully how her back had gotten so messed up when I walked out to her "car." My jaw dropped to my chest when I saw that she was driving a full-sized extended cab Ford F-350 pickup. My first thought was, "What? Is the dump truck in the shop?"

I've watched people mount skittish horses with greater ease than Lynn showed climbing up into the driver's seat.

Getting baby burrito, Jayden, strapped in safely took almost as much time and a lot more effort than Lynn's entire appointment. As I dropped back to the pavement in a bone-jarring move reminiscent of a skydiver landing, I decided that her mode of transportation would be a topic of conversation the next time Lynn was in the office.

It was obvious . . . She'd be back.

How can driving my baby around in an SUV be bad for my back?

You would probably be surprised by the sheer number of new moms who arrive at my office driving massive SUVs. I know it's a daily occurrence.

A sport-utility vehicle is built high off the ground. That means to get your baby in and out, you need to climb onto the running board then reach up and over to deposit or retrieve your baby from his or her car seat. The bigger the SUV, the greater the risk to your back. Your back has to go through all sorts of contortions just to deal with the design of your vehicle. And every twist and turn stresses your weakened joints and ligaments.

───────────

The bigger the SUV, the greater the risk to your back.

───────────

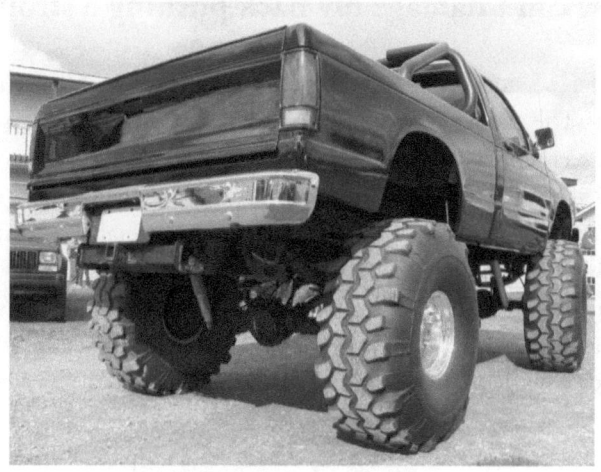

Remember, you only need to strain your back one time out of a zillion to cause long-term back pain.

As uncool as it sounds, the best vehicle for your back's health is the dreaded minivan. I acknowledge up front that minivans have an image issue. You are free, of course, to drive whatever vehicle you want. However, I would be remiss in pointing out the advantages minivans present for your back and neck health.

First, minivans are built lower to the ground than SUVs, so you can step in and out with very little effort and virtually no climbing. In most cases, you are level with your baby, rather than reaching up for him or her. The minivan also offers large no-swing doors, so there are no major twisting contortions to go through getting in or out. With some models, the doors slide open with a touch of a button.

You also don't risk jarring your spine every time you step down from the height of an SUV.

Lastly, you can't discount the vehicle's suspension: a minivan rides like a car, not like a truck. That's especially important to your low back over long car rides.

Every mother I know who is also a chiropractor, including my wife, drives a minivan. What they lose in coolness factor an hour or so every day, they more than make up for by avoiding backaches 24/7.

How can I damage my back pushing a stroller?

The good news is most people can push a stroller with confidence that their back isn't in jeopardy. The glaring exception is if the parent doing the pushing stands more than about five feet nine inches tall.

Because of the way most strollers are engineered, the handles are set for parents who are considered short to average in height. Anyone taller is forced to stretch and bend at the waist to engage the handles and push the stroller. Compounding the discomfort is the fact that a longer gait usually results in the tall stroller pusher impacting the axle of the stroller with his or her foot. If you look around the shopping mall, you'll undoubtedly see more than a few folks pushing a stroller who are hunched over, shuffling their feet.

If either you or your husband are tall, you'll need to shop for a stroller with a handle extension. This isn't a common feature, and you may be faced with the more cumbersome "jog stroller" to comfortably accommodate the pusher's height.

I recommend to all my patients that they try out the stroller in the store. You can check out the height of the handles, but you can also see whether the model you're considering requires you to bend at the waist in order to fold it up.

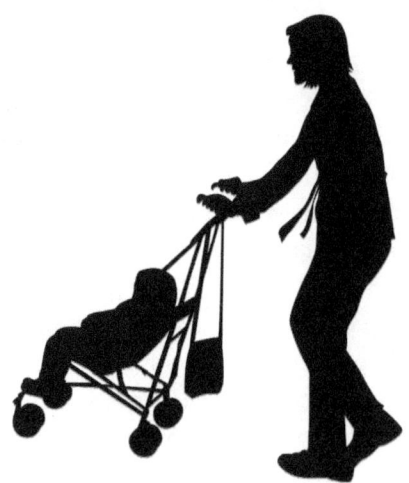

How can a baby carrier hurt my back?

Anything that puts strain on your back can lead to long-term back maladies.

There are a great many baby carriers on the market. The baby carriers I recommend are the ones that allow you to strap the baby very close to your chest. You want to choose one that is lightweight and allows for multiple positions. I'm not in the business of recommending specific brands of products, but I would suggest that you find one that is designed similar to the Weego brand that is currently on the market. From personal experience, I've found that particular design to be effective, safe, and versatile, with very little risk of back strain.

How can a crib hurt my back?

The ergonomic design of baby beds has improved over the years. The most important thing to remember with a newborn is to raise the mattress so you don't have to bend over to lift your baby out of the crib.

The safety of your baby isn't compromised with a high mattress until the little darling starts standing. By the time your baby stands, he or she has gotten fairly big. Lifting him or her out of the crib is potentially more dangerous to your back. Drop the side of the crib whenever possible. And lift with your knees bent to let your thighs do the lifting, not your back. Hold your baby close to your chest.

How can a changing table hurt my back?

When you change your baby on a changing table, you usually stand at the side of the table with your body positioned at a ninety-degree angle from your baby. "Sure," you respond. "What's wrong with that?"

If you are standing at the side of the changing table, you have to twist your body to actually change a diaper. Remember, your ligaments are hormonally loosened. When you twist your body to change the diaper, your back muscles have to compensate for the compromised ligaments.

When you twist your body to change the diaper, your back muscles have to compensate for the compromised ligaments.

Changing tables are great, but position yours so you can stand at the end of the table in line with your baby to change his or her diaper. Facing your baby with his or her feet facing toward you is the optimum position for your spine.

How can getting back in shape hurt my back?

I know that it is common for women to feel fat during and after pregnancy. Especially after giving birth, a large number of women want their old bodies back as soon as possible, and many see working out at the gym as the answer.

RUSH TO GET THIN

A patient I'll call Gayle came into my office for the first time three weeks after giving birth to her first child. Her complaint was low-back pain. In taking her history, I learned that she hadn't done stretches or exercises during her pregnancy. Once the baby was born, though, she decided to get into shape. Immediately.

Gayle went to a local gym and started jumping on the weight machines, determined to reclaim her figure. Using the heaviest weights she could handle, she did rotation exercises with resistance as well as trunk flexion with resistance.

The result was that she injured the connective tissues of the lumbar spine.

I have learned over my career that the worst question you can ever ask a patient is, "What were you thinking?" Guess what I asked Gayle.

We Americans almost always pump weights for strength. It's as though the more weight you can lift, the smarter, sexier, and better looking you become. Bull feathers. If you are currently weight training, my suggestion is to reduce the amount of weight and to increase the repetitions. The truth is strength and muscle tone can be accomplished with less taxing exercises and greater frequency. Be consistent.

Also, I urge you to seek the advice of a trained physical therapist before you hit the weight room or start any kind of exercise routine in your postpartum condition.

How can a pillow help my back?

Pillows are a great invention for managing back discomfort.

A body pillow is great for sleeping with your body aligned while on your side. This is a great tool while you are pregnant as well as after the birth of your baby.

I also recommend a nursing pillow for taking the stress off your upper back and neck while feeding your baby. A properly designed pillow will allow you to hold your baby higher and closer without straining your muscles.

I also recommend a nursing pillow for taking the stress off your upper back and neck while feeding your baby.

In my practice, I have seen that lap or nursing pillows greatly decrease the chance of postpartum neck and midback pain.

One trick my wife discovered is to always place a pillow vertically in your nursing chair to add support to your midback. After she showed me the technique, I noticed that at the hospital, the good nurses always used the same system for new moms.

CHAPTER 15

YOUR NECK AND HEADACHES (PART 2)

How am I still at risk for neck pain and headaches after I've given birth?

Often, the culprit is your enlarged breasts. The man in your life will probably be quite enthusiastic when your postpartum breasts balloon to *Playboy* Playmate-like proportions. That's because we men are idiots. We start practicing being stupid in this area when we're about thirteen, and we master the behavior by about eighteen.

Unfortunately, the enlargement of your breasts as they fill with milk can develop upper-back tension in many women. The extra pulling forward of the added weight may cause muscle discomfort and tingling in one or both of your arms and hands.

Typically, though, women can adjust to the increased size of their breasts. A sensible mechanical aid is to wear a new supportive, well-fitting bra that gives you support to combat the downward pull.

How can breast-feeding cause neck pain and headaches?

Frequently, you're as much to blame as your breasts for causing back pain and its accompanying headaches. It occurs because of the flexion of the neck while the baby is feeding.

Come feeding time, your maternal instinct takes over, and you become enthralled watching your baby feed at your breast. Your head bends forward in an awkward position, and your neck stresses. You can spend hours a day in this position, and your neck will be worse for wear.

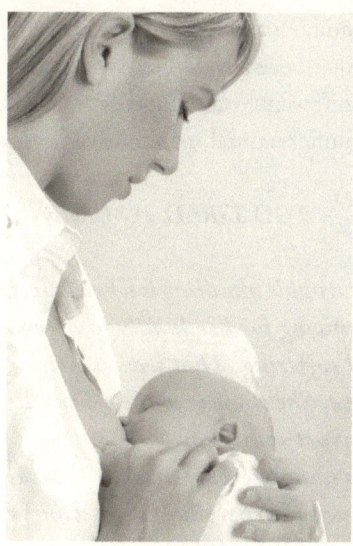

The way you would like to feed your baby.
It often leads to neck pain.

When you breast-feed, tip your head back once the little one gets the latching part down. This will help you enjoy your baby even more because you'll have less neck discomfort and fewer headaches. Also, place a pillow long ways behind your back while you're feeding. Remember again back to the days just after you gave birth: this is the technique the nurses advocated when you first started to feed your baby.

What does thoracic outlet syndrome mean to my neck and head?

Thoracic outlet syndrome or *TOS* sounds terrible, but is basically just peripheral nerve and vessel entrapment or compression syndrome over the upper back, neck, and shoulder involving bone and muscles. Peripheral entrapment is a medical way of describing when the nerves and blood vessels are being pinched by structures away from the spine.

There are three different TOSs depending on which structures are doing the compressing. All of the TOS conditions are differentiated by orthopedic testing. They must also be distinguished from nerve root compression in the neck.

The three TOS conditions are as follows:

1. *scalene anticus syndrome*—what I like to call "smushed-up organ syndrome"
2. *claviculocostal syndrome*—which I call "enlarged-breast syndrome"
3. *pectoralis minor syndrome*—what I refer to as "car seat back"

Understanding these conditions and where they occur is important to proper treatment. After the baby is born and you notice any of these symptoms, have them checked out by a doctor of chiropractic. You don't want to take unnecessary medications while breast-feeding, and a good chiropractor can offer natural, noninvasive treatments.

TOO TIRED TO CARE

The type of case I have trouble handling is when a patient comes in for temporary relief and is too busy sacrificing for her family to do what's necessary to eliminate the cause of the pain and suffering. That was exactly what happened with a new mom whom we'll call Sonya. She came into the office with her eight-month-old son, Randy, a beautiful and robust young boy.

At the time, Sonya was twenty-seven years old. As I was taking her medical history and looking at Randy, who never left her side, I started thinking that the timing was right for neck pain and headaches, classic TOS (thoracic outlet syndrome) symptoms.

Before Sonya even told me when Randy had been born, I had done the math and determined his age based on his size. I asked about the labor and push time.

When she finally got to listing her reasons for seeing me, I already knew what they'd be: neck pain accompanied by upper-back referral pain along with some headaches.

With the history out of the way, I started the actual exam. It quickly became apparent her neck and upper-back conditions didn't develop overnight but had been building over a period of at least several months.

Although I suspected the answer, I asked Sonya if she had had any massage or chiropractic care pregnancy during her pregnancy with Randy. As I predicted, the answer was a resounding no.

My first reaction was that she needed a massage stat! *(That's doctor talk for "no time to wait.") Sonya's neck was a complete mess.*

I was confident that if we had worked with Sonya throughout her pregnancy, most, if not all, of her current aches and pains could have been avoided. Sadly, I knew Sonya before she got pregnant, and I couldn't help but notice how exhausted and frazzled she looked.

Throughout our visit, Sonya had been trying to entertain and distract Randy with her car keys and whatever else she found handy. As clever and as insightful as I had been, it was obvious that she really wasn't paying much attention to me. She was consumed with little Randy. She was so tired from living on four hours' sleep—between her maternal duties and her work schedule—that nothing I said was getting through to her.

What this once-vibrant, vivacious woman needed was some "me" time without Randy in the room. She needed a massage or two, a couple of spinal adjustments, and a couple of dinners out.

What I wanted to do was call her husband and tell him to come get his son while his wife spent some time getting a massage. What I did was work on her neck and upper back as best I could with the constant presence of Randy fussing in the background.

As Sonya was leaving, she couldn't schedule a follow-up appointment because she was unable to predict when she might be free to come back. I suspected I wouldn't see her until the pain became unbearable again.

I had done the best I could under the circumstances; only I knew I hadn't done nearly enough to relieve Sonya's pain.

"Smushed-up" organ syndrome.

One of the three thoracic outlet syndromes called *scalene anticus syndrome* is a common condition with pregnancy and even after the baby is born. The symptoms include pain over the top of the shoulders to the neck on one or both sides. Symptoms can also include hands and fingers that are "going to sleep" or the sensation of "pins and needles" into the hands. These symptoms are usually most notable in the middle of the night or in early morning.

You will most likely have "aching" over one or both arms.

In pregnant women, this syndrome generally manifests itself in the late second trimester or early third trimester when all of your organs are smashed up against your lungs, making breathing more of an adventure.

Your body, sensing the need for oxygen, will work extra hard to force air into your lungs, constantly elevating your ribs (including your first rib) with as much force as possible. This will cause excessive pulling on the scalene attachment to your first and second ribs, causing elevation of these ribs with any neck movement or even a breath.

This is also the technical explanation for the neck pain associated with breast-feeding that we've discussed previously. After you have stressed your neck with labor, you tend to want to watch the baby while he or she eats.

Treatment for this syndrome include the following:

- ♦ massage to relax contracted muscles
- ♦ chiropractic treatment to reduce the first/second rib subluxation
- ♦ stretch front of neck and shoulders—wall stretch exercise
- ♦ home traction unit for neck

Enlarged-breast syndrome.

As mentioned earlier, your bigger breasts can cause some mechanical complications. This condition is the second type of thoracic outlet syndrome condition, *claviculocostal syndrome.*

This generally occurs after pregnancy when the nerves and vessels, the neurovascular bundle, is compressed between the clavicle (collarbone) and the first rib (costal). It gets its technical name because of the two bones involved in the compression.

The symptoms are similar to *scalene anticus syndrome*, but the sensation is best described as a weakness rather than a tingling of the hands and arms, and *claviculocostal syndrome* is usually experienced after your milk comes in due to the downward pulling of your bra straps over your shoulders due to the weight of your enlarged breasts.

Treatment for *claviculocostal syndrome* is the same as *scalene anticus syndrome.*

Car seat back.

The third thoracic outlet syndrome is called *pectoralis minor syndrome*. It shows up about twelve to eighteen months after the birth and is usually caused by lifting and carrying the baby and, most often, from the unusual strain you put on your pectoralis (chest) muscles from leaning in and situating or removing your child from his or her car seat.

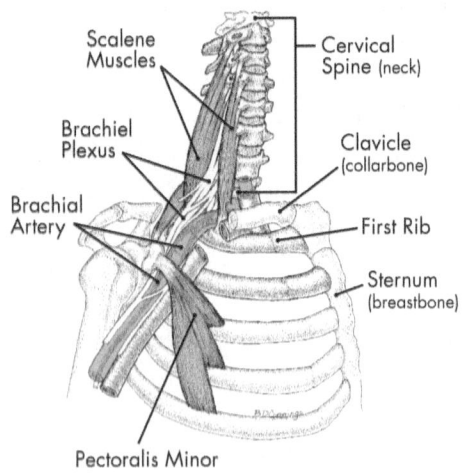

All three TOSs involve these anatomical structures.

Symptoms are essentially the same as the other two forms of TOS, including numbness and weakness in the hands with an achy sensation in the neck and over the shoulders.

The syndrome is defined from compression of the neurovascular bundle between the pectoralis minor muscle, a thin triangular muscle situated at the upper part of the chest, and the rib cage. With this syndrome, the brachial nerve and axillary artery and vein become compressed under the pectoralis minor muscle.

As your baby gets heavier, it is your deep chest muscle that has to continually compensate. Over time, it becomes overworked and can compress the neurovascular components under it.

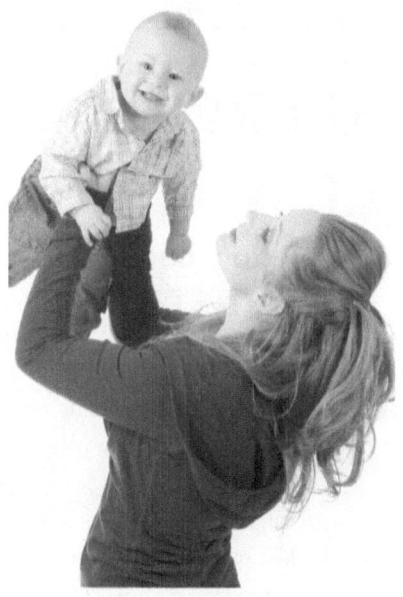

You're encouraged to play with your baby, of course.
This position, though, can lead to TOS.

Treatment for this syndrome is similar to the other forms of TOS with the exception that the chiropractor will actually work somewhat lower on your rib cage and spine. This type of TOS responds well to stretching exercises.

CHAPTER 16

YOUR RECOVERY

What can I do to get my body back to how it was before I got pregnant?

After forty weeks of dramatic changes in your body, hormonal modifications, notable weight gain, ligament loosening, and muscle adjustments, your body must now resume a semblance of its former self. This is important for your back health as well as your general well-being.

You need to put in some work to protect your back after your baby's birth. It's time to enlist the help of some of the key members of your back health care team—your chiropractor, your massage therapist, your physical therapist, and your nutritionist.

How can I get into good shape quickly?

My advice: lose the word *quickly* from your mind-set. Don't try to lose weight too rapidly or tone your body overnight. Be realistic. It took you nine months to get your body where it is today. It's not unreasonable to predict that it will take you at least that amount of time to get back to the shape you were in before you got pregnant. A slow, steady pace is important because you aren't just losing weight—your body is recovering from the rigors of pregnancy and childbirth.

My advice: lose the word quickly *from your mind-set.*

I know that you've seen photographs of actresses and other celebrities on the covers of magazines shortly after they've given birth. They appear slim, elegant, fashionable, and sexy. You'd never guess from the shot that the woman pictured was a new mom. In the article on the inside of the publication, she may even brag about the exercise regimen she started with her personal trainer the day she got home from the hospital. Baloney. Don't fall for it. She's trying to stay in the limelight and get back to work as soon as possible.

Even if someone is willing to pay you several million dollars for three months' work, movie star money, the risk to your health and your baby's just isn't worth it.

The movie star message is that you must do all you can do to become as thin as possible as quickly as possible after your baby is born. That philosophy is both ludicrous and unhealthy. The weeks and months right after you've given birth are challenging, taxing both your physical and emotional strength. I'm all for your eating sensibly, but losing weight shouldn't be the focus of your diet.

Your diet should be *low fat*, but not *fat free*. It should be vitamin rich and high in fiber. Whatever you do, don't get tricked into trying a fad diet. You run the risk of actually slowing down your recovery process if you deprive your metabolism of essential nutrients by loading or avoiding things like protein and carbohydrates.

Work with your nutritionist to make sure you get a proper balance of protein, fresh vegetables, and dairy products. Avoid fast foods and things like processed meats.

Keep in mind that you need to consume at least eighteen hundred calories a day while you're breast-feeding in order to stay healthy and keep your baby nourished properly. Check with your nutritionist for menu suggestions and dos and don'ts.

How can breast-feeding help me get back in shape?

This is great news. Not only is breast-feeding good for your baby, the American College of Obstetricians and Gynecologists has reported that breast-feeding leads to the release of hormones that enable your uterus to return to its normal size.

Breast-feeding leads to the release of hormones that enable your uterus to return to its normal size.

What kinds of exercises can I do?

As you can imagine, there are lots of reasons to exercise during the months after you've given birth. Obviously, a combination of proper diet and exercise can help you lose weight faster and get into shape. Remember, it won't be long before you're running all over the house, chasing after a little lively toddler.

I recommend that you develop a workout regimen with your physical therapist with the dual goals of helping you lose weight and of strengthening the muscles in your back and pelvis.

Physical activity has also been shown to be a great way to combat postpartum depression, improve your emotional outlook, and boost your confidence. My wife explains that it's a great way to *clear her head* so she's better able to focus on the demands of being a mom.

Physical activity has also been shown to be a great way to combat postpartum depression, improve your emotional outlook, and boost your confidence.

Gina is an advocate of joining Mommy & Me exercise classes that let your baby exercise along with you. Not only do you get a workout, you get to interact with other moms who are facing the same issues you deal with every day.

An added benefit of physical activity is that it gives you increased energy, something you'll need lots of over the next few years.

How can suddenly losing weight hurt my back?

First of all, I realize that *you* are far from average. But for the sake of this discussion, I'll refer to averages.

The average weight gain during pregnancy is twenty-five to thirty-five pounds, or 11.34-15.88 kilograms. Again, that's an average; your actual weight gain can be higher or lower.

Let's say your baby weighs seven and a half pounds, or 3.4 kilograms. The amniotic fluid, placenta, and extra body fluids in your body are another eight to twelve pounds, or 3.63-5.44 kilograms. The moment you give birth, your weight is reduced immediately by about fourteen pounds, or 6.35 kilograms, which can be half of your total weight gain.

In other words, much of the weight you gained during pregnancy will be gone shortly after you give birth. Your ligaments will still be loose, and your muscles will need to adjust to the dramatic shift in your center of gravity. You might want to go back and read chapter 6, "Your Posture."

It just makes sense that you are susceptible to back injury when you factor in the data that you're now carrying around an eight-pound wiggling weight in your arms.

I recommend that you get some hands-on work with your chiropractor and especially your massage therapist once a week to help reestablish your center of gravity through neurological receptor feedback. Investing a little money on mommy's well-being will pay dividends for the whole family, including baby and ol' what's-his-name.

CHAPTER 17

YOUR PERFECT BABY

As I alluded to earlier in this book, short push times are a good thing.

For moms, a short push time means less time in labor. Physically, that translates to less lumbar flexion and less intra-abdominal pressures where disc damage can occur.

For babies, an expedited birth is a terrific birthday present. With quick passage through the birth canal, the head will take its proper shape much more quickly, and neck trauma is typically avoided.

For babies, an expedited birth is a terrific birthday present.

Most folks ask about the baby's gender, length, and weight. I always ask about push times. What can I say? I'm just a sentimental fool. I also check the baby's head for angel kisses and stork bites. (It's a doctor thing; don't try it at home.)

How can a long push time make my baby colicky?

Long push times can translate into potential long-term problems resulting from neck trauma and lopsided head. Babies who have spent an inordinately long period of time in the birth canal tend to suffer upper-alignment issues of the neck, specifically C1 and C2. (You might want to check appendix A for an explanation of the cervical spine.)

Remember, your baby has exactly the same spine structure that you have, subject to the same stresses, strains, and pains.

"Alignment problems in my brand-new baby?" you challenge. "Preposterous!"

As much as we want our babies to be perfect when they are born, the reality is their first activity is both strenuous and traumatic. My wife has given birth four times, and I know from experience that it isn't an easy experience for anyone involved.

Over the years, many moms have come to me with colicky babies. Often, a pediatrician will explain that the condition is the result of an underdeveloped digestive system or declare the malady a *pyloric sphincter* (stomach opening) problem and prescribe baby antacids because the little darling is vomiting. Many times, antacids don't do the trick.

Since the baby is throwing up, it's obviously a stomach problem. Right?

Not necessarily. Having seen several births live and in living color, I can confirm that the baby's head goes through several contortions and that the doctor at some point is going to grab the head, which makes up about a third of your baby's body, and possibly pull. Possibly pull really hard.

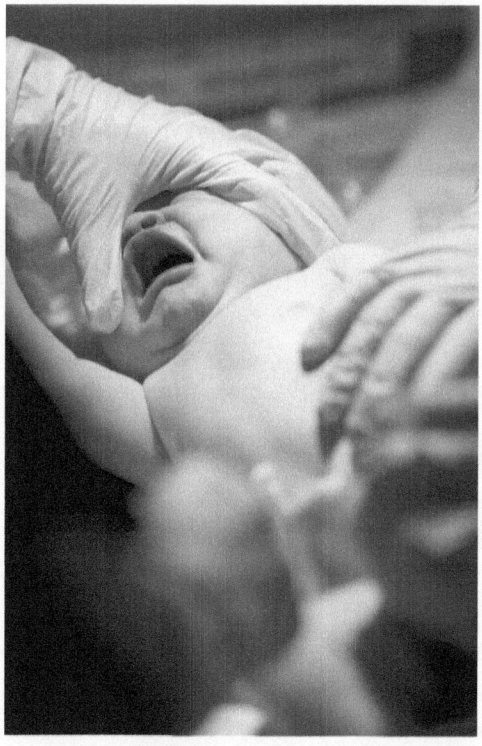

Maybe, instead of a bellyache, your baby has a headache. How does your baby tell you that his or her stomach hurts? He or she cries. How does your baby communicate a pain in the head? He or she cries. How can you differentiate one from the other? I don't know, and I've had four kids and treated hundreds more.

"But," in your best Sherlock Holmes mode you counter, "my baby is projectile vomiting. It has to be a stomach problem!"

Maybe.

Have you ever suffered from motion sickness in a car, boat, or plane? Have you ever had a headache that made you nauseous?

Many children suffer from upper-neck alignment problems after birth due to the ordeal of being born. They feel intense pain (as we would in their shoes or booties) and suffer from headaches and, possibly, vertigo and dizziness.

They hurt. They cry. They throw up.

Many children suffer from upper-neck alignment problems after birth due to the ordeal of being born.

THE STORY OF BABY LEO

Baby Leo's mother, Mary Ann, was coming to me for lower-back pain and neck issues. I couldn't help but notice that she was fatigued, worn out, and tired. I asked her what was wrong.

She looked at me with sad eyes and explained that her newborn, little Leo, was on a sudden infant death syndrome (SIDS) monitor because he struggled with his breathing and that the monitor was going off virtually every hour. Leo was in distress, and Mary Ann was just plain stressed.

I asked whether she had Leo with her that day, and when she said yes, I humbly asked if I could see him.

As soon as she brought the little guy into my office, I noticed that he had a very lopsided head. It was instantly obvious. That observation naturally caused me to ask the troubled mom about her pregnancy and delivery.

As I suspected, baby Leo came into the world reluctantly, requiring a tug-of-war head pull.

I asked Mary Ann if it would be okay for me to examine and treat her treasure. When she agreed, I gently corrected his upper-cervical vertebrae, which had been significantly rotated during the birthing process.

I explained that her brave little man would most likely whimper but should experience a much better night's sleep. I saw hope in Mary Ann's eyes, but I knew she was also a little skeptical; that happens a lot when corrections look a little too easy. To ease her anxiety, I went on to explain the physiology behind the mechanical adjustments I had made.

The next day, I got a phone call from Leo's mom. She was crying.

Concerned, I asked her what had happened.

"The SIDS monitor didn't go off one time last night," she explained through her tears. "He slept the whole night without waking up!"

A high-tech SIDS monitor lost its job after that day.

Today, Mary Ann is one of my favorite patients, and she's expecting her fifth child. She comes to me before, during, and after each pregnancy; and I have examined each of her babies shortly after birth.

I still see Leo from time to time. He has grown into a fine little boy with a bright future.

I am continually amazed by how quickly people jump to the conclusion that a spinal correction by a licensed professional chiropractor can be harmful yet accept without question the potential side effects of prescribed medication for their children. I guess it's a combination of the lack of stature of doctors of chiropractic in the medical community in general coupled with the fact that there's never been a good chiropractor show on prime-time television although there's a chiropractor character on a current TV sitcom—he's not exactly portrayed as the second coming of George Clooney's Dr. Doug Ross on *ER*, and we don't see him helping people in pain on a weekly basis.

Have I ever failed to successfully treat a colicky baby with chiropractic? Of course. Some kids actually do have abdominal and digestive tract issues. Sometimes, they're born with ailments; and sometimes, their stomach complaints are the result of long-term use of antacids that have, in some cases, permanently altered the digestive organs.

If your chiropractor has specific expertise in infants—please check to make sure they do—he or she can examine your newborn and help determine whether the *colic* is stomach related or due to cervical misalignment.

As a dad who deeply loves his own kids, I always consider it the highest possible honor when I'm asked to examine someone else's baby.

It has been my clinical experience that kids born with short push times tend to avoid neck and cervical spine problems.

THE NEARLY PERFECT PREGNANCY

I know, perfection is something we can only strive toward but never achieve. Still . . .

A mother-to-be who—we'll call her Molly—was urged to see me by her husband, Jerry who has been a patient for a few years. Molly is an attractive woman in her midtwenties, and she was pregnant with their first baby. She is also nearly six feet tall.

Jerry is also quite tall.

Molly and Jerry gave all the signs of a storybook marriage. They obviously care deeply for each other, and they were in full agreement that they were going to do everything within their power for her pregnancy and their baby.

When Molly visited my office for her first appointment, I could see that she was already in very good physical shape. I learned that she is quite proficient at yoga and has a longtime commitment to good nutrition. In fact, throughout her pregnancy, whenever I asked about food concerns, she was right on target, especially with her protein intake.

Never missing an appointment, Molly was diligent with every aspect of her body. Exercises and stretches? No problem. Admittedly, she had some backaches we had to deal with over the course of the pregnancy; but overall, she did well with treatments. Molly was as close to a perfect patient as any prenatal chiropractor could ask for.

As time went on, it became evident that Molly was getting quite large. If you can visualize a nearly six-foot-tall tummy, you get the idea.

Jerry's mother, Marie, has also been a patient of mine for many years. One day in passing, I asked her how big Jerry was when he was born. The answer: over ten pounds. I didn't need years of clinical experience to know that Molly's baby was going to be a bruiser when he or she came into the world.

Molly's preparation and commitment to following doctor's orders made her a textbook case. All systems were go by the time the big day came.

Shortly after the birth, Molly and Jerry came into my office proudly carrying their baby in a car seat. Sitting in the seat was Justin, a beautiful little smiling red-headed boy who really wasn't very little. Justin's features were perfectly symmetrical, so I naturally asked about the birth, expecting to hear about a textbook delivery with a short push time.

I was genuinely surprised to learn that Molly required an emergency caesarean section. It turns out that the baby was over nine pounds and refused to come out the pelvic outlet. I knew that avoiding a C-section was one of Molly's prime motivators.

Molly's pelvis was aligned, her nutrition was good, and she was in great shape. We did everything right.

Instead of questioning why or who could have done what, Molly was at peace with the result. She had the maturity and strength to understand that there are just some things that are out of our control. What a healthy attitude!

As Molly expressed to me, at the end of the day, she and Jerry had a wonderful new life in their family.

The lesson here, and the reason I've included Molly's story in this book, is to remind every reader that the main reason for working hard for nine months is to bring a healthy, bouncing bundle of joy into the world. Even when everything doesn't go the way we'd like, the outcome is still going to call you Mommy and change your life forever.

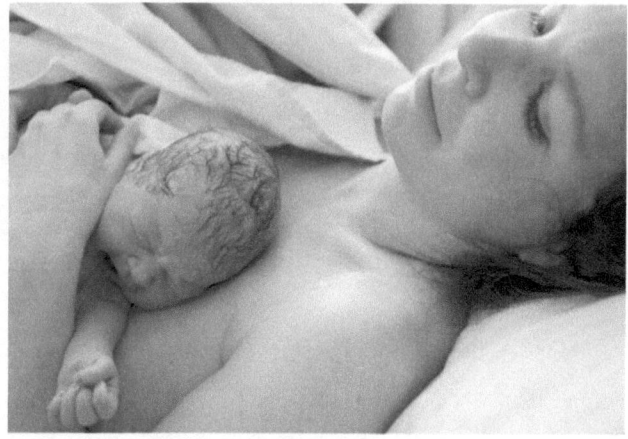

APPENDIX A

THE ANATOMY OF YOUR BACK

In order for body movement to occur, the back is comprised of a complex assembly incorporating multiple bones as well as discs, joints, ligaments, muscles, and nerves.

Here is an illustration of the components of your back:

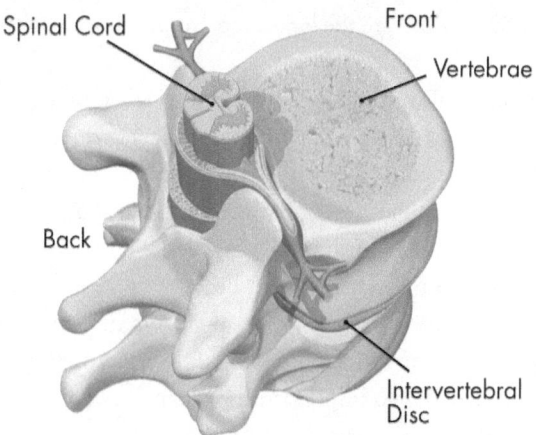

Vertebrae.

The spine is comprised of thirty-three vertebrae, twenty-four of which are mobile—cervical, thoracic, and lumbar—and nine are fused, immobile structures that make up the sacrum and the coccyx.

The upper three regions are grouped under the names *cervical* (seven vertebrae), *thoracic* (twelve vertebrae) and *lumbar* (five vertebrae). To these twenty-four vertebrae, which are each separated by intervertebral discs, are added the nine vertebrae at the bottom of the column, five vertebrae that are fused to form the *sacrum* and four *coccygeal* bones that form the *tailbone*.

The moveable vertebrae are donut-shaped interlocking bones approximately one inch tall. They are stacked one upon the other like a column. The spinal column gives your back structure. It also houses and protects ten billion nerve cells in the delicate and vital structure known as the spinal cord.

Facet joints.

Between the vertebrae are small gliding joints called facet joints. Each vertebra has four facets, two above and two below. These small joints control the angles in which your spine moves. Irritation and inflammation of these joints result in back pain. It is not unreasonable to assume that, in many women, carrying the baby's weight can create just such an inflammation.

Intervertebral discs.

To give the spinal column freedom of movement, discs are located between the vertebrae. The discs comprise about a third of the length of the spine and function as natural shock absorbers. The discs are made up of two parts, a gelatinous center called the *nucleus pulposus* and a tough radial tirelike outer covering made up of interwoven cartilage. Collectively, the discs are the largest organs of the body without its own blood supply.

A disc gets virtually all of its nourishment through a process called imbibition, fluid movement from the *nucleus pulposus* through the vertebral end plates. As the day progresses, your discs gradually push water out of the *nucleus pulposus*. It is precisely this mechanism that causes you to be a quarter of an inch shorter at the end of the day than when you woke up in the morning.

This is significant to a pregnant woman because the loss of fluid creates a higher load on the discs. If too much pressure is put on a disc, it can compress and become ruptured or herniated, causing significant pain while undermining the integrity of the spinal column. That's why it's so important for pregnant women to lie down and rest for short periods throughout the day.

Ligaments.

Along with the vertebrae, joints, and discs, your spine has ligaments. They are long flexible strands of an elastic, fibrous tissue that resemble rubber bands. Their function is to hold the vertebral bones together, stabilize the spine, and protect the discs. The ligaments come in a variety of lengths and widths and help support and buttress the vertebrae while protecting the spinal column against jarring and sudden heavy blows.

Muscles.

Hundreds of muscles in the back move and support the spine. The familiar "soft tissue" injury to the back often involves these muscles. In fact, doctors diagnose "nonspecific backache" for 56 percent of the patients who come to them with low-back pain.

THE ANATOMY OF YOUR POSTURE

As we saw back in chapter 4, what we would call *bad* posture has the very real potential of creating back pain. Especially during pregnancy, you need to be cognizant of your posture and to work hard to maintain proper body positioning at all times to minimize the stress and resultant discomfort on your spinal column.

Attaining good posture is a little more complex than your mom yelling "Stand up straight!" whenever you slouch.

In the medical community, there are two widely recognized concepts of posture: the *developmental* concept of posture and the *neurological* model of posture.

THE DEVELOPMENTAL CONCEPT OF POSTURE

We'll discuss the *developmental concept of posture* first. This concept notes that posture in an adult is related to three factors: (1) heredity, (2) disease, and (3) acquired habit.

Hereditary posture: This part of the concept indicates that people have a genetic posture that comes from their mom and dad. The truth is people come in all shapes and sizes. Look to your mom and dad to see what your future looks like if you just continue with your posture as it is today. In my clinical experience, I have observed that you have either your mom's or your dad's spine, rarely a mixture of the two. I'm convinced that you can do something about improving your posture.

If someone is heavy or big boned or exceptionally tall, for example, your body type will obviously impact your posture.

I have found with my patients that changing diet, exercise, and sleep patterns can actually improve a hereditary-posture situation. To effect this change requires thoughtful, conscious effort.

Disease posture: People suffer from several posture-affecting diseases that are too many to list here, but include things like *rheumatoid arthritis, ankylosing spondylitis,* and pathological *scoliosis,* among others. *Subluxated* (nonmoving) joints in a young child, if left untreated, can also affect posture long term.

Acquired posture: This is the impact our environment has on your posture. Sometimes, we mimic the posture of those we admire. Also, we all acquire postural changes due to work, relaxation, home furnishings, sports activities, recreation, culture, diet, and, for the female segment of the population, pregnancy. Our environment can be difficult to change. If you sit eight hours a day at a computer keyboard, your pregnant body is going to have an effect on your posture.

THE NEUROLOGICAL CONCEPT OF POSTURE

In order for you to fully understand what I'm going to be describing as the neurological concept of posture, I'm first going to have to give you a brief anatomy lesson. I'll try to make it as painless as possible, but you may need a nap partway through.

First, here's what your spinal column looks like:

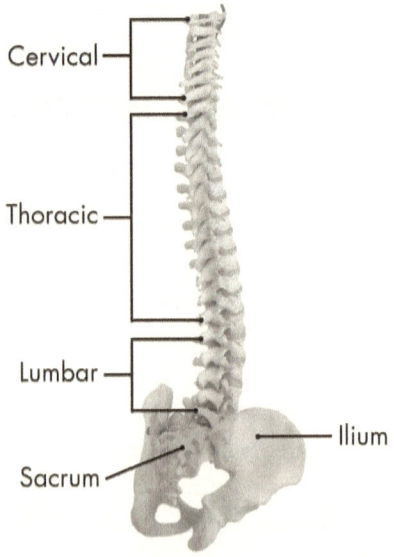

The vertebral column has four basic curves:

1. The cervical (neck) curvature is *lordotic*. That's a medical term that means it bends concave to the posterior. *Lordisus*, from the Greek for "bent backward," is a medical term used to describe an inward curvature of a portion of the vertebral column. Two segments of the vertebral column, both the cervical and lumbar, are *normally* lordotic; that is, they are set in a curve that has its convexity in front and concavity behind.
2. The thoracic (midback) curvature is *kyphotic* or convex toward the back. *Kyphosis*, from the Greek for "bent," is a rearward curvature of the spinal column.
3. The lumbar (lower-back) curvature is lordotic or concave to the posterior.
4. The sacral (tailbone) curvature is convex to the posterior.

Those are the curves. Now you're probably wondering how a bony part of your body can change the shape of curves. The reason was presented in appendix A: The spinal column is not solid bone but is made up of many *vertebrae* of different sizes. These individual irregular bones of your spinal column allow it to change its curvature.

The default mechanism of the *neurologic concept of posture* calls for the muscle tension along the vertical axis of the spine to be regulated by brain and sensory neurons.

Your body continually makes adjustments without you even thinking about it. The problem with being pregnant, though, is that the size, shape, and movement of the baby dictates that you may, in effect, need to manually override the system.

The process is initiated when the sensory neurons send *proprioceptive* impulses from the body's peripheral nerves through the spinal column to inform the body of its relationship to the center of gravity.

Your body automatically senses where your center of gravity is. This becomes complicated with a pregnant woman, though, because your center of gravity is continually changing—not just month to month, but minute to minute and even hearbeat to heartbeat.

The spinal joints (explained in appendix A) most responsible for the proprioception or feedback are found, ironically, in the spine where lower-back pain is manifested.

When the message is received by your brain, it in turn sends impulses out to the ligaments, joint capsules, skin, viscera, and muscle attachments from your feet, knees, and hips to compensate for the change in your center of gravity.

The *vestibular system* controls balance. It is located in the inner ear and coordinates the compensating reflexes of the eyes and head. This automatic response mechanism is responsible for keeping your eyes level with the horizon. It also sends input to the central nervous system informing the body of the center of gravity.

Medically speaking, pressure variants, nociceptive sensations, movements, and touch sensations are sent to the central nervous system to the medulla, which constantly and instantaneously sends back messages to the appropriate body parts controlling posture.

The constant change in spinal curvatures with shifting weight and a rapidly shifting center of gravity continually alters the proprioception of your spinal structure. While all of that is happening, the cortical (high-brain) function must accept the input as "feeling normal." Often, the result is an expectant mother who is complaining about "bad posture" and backache.

APPENDIX C

THE ANATOMY OF YOUR PELVIS

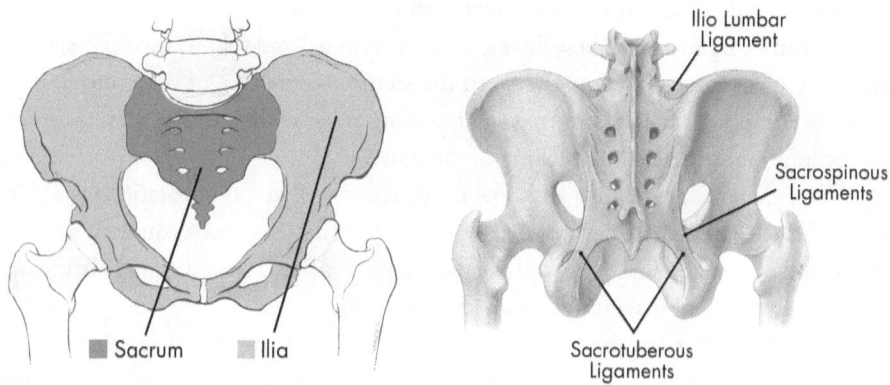

Structure.

Your pelvis is made up of two bones called *ilia* (shown in purple) that are connected by cartilage called the *pubis symphysis*.

The *sacrum* (shown in orange) is comprised of five fused vertebrae. It bridges the ilia together.

You probably call the coccyx (shown in green) your tailbone. It is connected to the sacrum with a bunch of small ligaments.

Most ligament groups of the pelvis are named for the bones they connect.

Hormones.

The hormone *relaxin* is released in later pregnancy to encourage pelvic ligaments, as well as the cervix and pelvic muscles, to loosen up and become very elastic. Your pelvis is working extra hard to support your trunk during pregnancy, yet relaxin is compromising the ligaments at the same time. The hormone effectively causes additional contracture and pressure on the core muscles of your spine.

As mentioned in the chapter on posture, this added demand on the muscles of the lower back and pelvis can be the source of pain throughout the last two trimesters of your pregnancy.

Ligaments.

Iliolumbar ligaments. Shown in green in the illustration below, these ligaments are responsible for stabilizing and tethering the lower lumbar vertebrae to the pelvis (the ilium). When these ligaments become hormonally loosened, their ability to tether the lumbar spine is compromised due to the *hyperlordosis* of the lumbar spine. This is most noticeable when you try to stand your pregnant body back up after bending at the waist. In order to pull your body upright, the muscles in your lower back must be used for the task, often causing lower-back pain.

Sacroiliac ligaments. These ligaments (shown in red and yellow) establish stability of the sacroiliac joint—the joint between the sacrum, at the base of the spine, and the ilium of the pelvis. It is a strong weight-bearing joint with irregular elevations and depressions that produce interlocking of the bones.

The ligaments prevent up and down slippage as well as aid in rotational stability. When these ligaments become hormonally loosened during pregnancy, you are susceptible to rotation of the sacroiliac joint and the pain that's associated with it. This is frequently experienced with pubis symphysis pain as well.

These ligaments line both the front and the back of the sacroiliac joints. When you experience pain in these ligaments, you'll describe the area of discomfort as "high hip."

Sacrospinous and *sacrotuberous ligaments.* Together with the greater and lesser sciatic notches, they form the greater and lesser sciatic foramen. Although these two ligaments don't have direct contact with the hip joint, they are important in maintaining pelvic integrity. They also serve as landmarks when studying the relative positions of the pelvis and gluteal region.

The *sacrospinous* ligament extends from the ischial spine and the lower sacrum and coccyx, converting the greater sciatic notch into the greater sciatic foramen. The greater sciatic foramen is a conduit from the pelvis to the buttock and is divided in half by the piriformis muscle.

The *sacrotuberous* ligament extends from the sacrum to the ischial tuberosity converting the lesser sciatic notch into the lesser sciatic foramen. The lesser sciatic foramen is also a conduit to the perineum from the buttock for the pudendal nerves and vessels.

When these two ligaments are loosened in the third trimester of pregnancy, we see the sacral apex rotate to the posterior with an increase in anterior body weight.

The ilium also tends to close at the pelvic brim, creating tautness over the *sacrospinous* and *sacrotuberous* ligaments. When this happens, the greater sciatic foramen; and to a lesser extent, the lesser sciatic foramen become smaller. In the case of the greater sciatic foramen, this reduction in size causes undue stretching of the piriformis muscle, causing compression of the sciatic nerve. *This condition is known as piriformis syndrome.*

The medical dictionary definition of *piriformis syndrome* is "a neuromuscular disorder that occurs when the sciatic nerve is compressed or otherwise irritated by the piriformis muscle." The result is pain, tingling and numbness in the buttocks and along the course of the sciatic nerve—the back of the thigh, back of the leg, and even to the foot. It has long been believed that piriformis syndrome is the result of anatomical variations in the muscle-nerve relationship when the sciatic nerve becomes pinched between deep rotators of the hip.

In my clinical experience, piriformis syndrome occurs most frequently in women. In my opinion, the root cause of the condition is loosened ligaments during pregnancy resulting in true peripheral nerve entrapment.

GLOSSARY

To further your understanding of back pain in pregnancy, here is a listing of many of the words that have appeared in this book or that are often used in back pain and pregnancy discussions.

articular processes: Bony joints

cervical: The part of the spine between the head and the first rib (C1 through C7). This area is more commonly know as the neck.

chiropractic: A system of therapeutics based on the theory that disease is caused by interference with nerve function. A doctor of chiropractic restores the body to its normal condition by adjusting body structures, especially the spinal column.

coccygodynia: Damage to or breakage of the coccyx, the tailbone.

contraindication: A condition or factor that increases the *risks* involved in using a particular *drug*, carrying out a medical procedure, or engaging in a particular activity.

disc: The rubbery structure, shaped like a jelly donut, which separates one spinal vertebra from another, adding flexibility and shock-absorbing qualities to the spine. Like a jelly donut, the outer layer of the disc is made of multiple-sized layers of strong ligament tissue with the center filled with a gelatinous material that responds to the varying stresses and pressures that are exerted on the spinal column.

doula: *Doula* is a Greek word that means "women's servant." Women have been serving other women in childbirth for centuries. In today's culture, a doula is a professional who is trained in childbirth and provides emotional, physical, and informational support to a woman who is expecting, in labor, or has recently given birth.

dystocia: An abnormal or difficult childbirth or labor. Dystocia may arise due to incoordinate uterine activity, abnormal fetal lie or presentation, or absolute or relative cephalopelvic disproportion.

ectopic: An ectopic pregnancy is one in which the fertilized egg is implanted in any tissue other than the uterine wall. Most ectopic pregnancies occur in the fallopian tube (so-called tubal pregnancies); but implantation can also occur in the cervix, ovaries, and abdomen.

edema: Formerly known as *dropsy* or *hydropsy*, edema is the increase of interstitial fluid in any organ.

facet joints: Tiny joints that link spinal vertebrae; each vertebra has four facets, two above and two below.

herniated disc: The damaged or broken surface of the disc that separates spinal vertebrae; also commonly referred to as a *slipped disc*, a *ruptured disc*, or a *herniated nucleus pulposus (HNP)*.

hormones: A *hormone* is a chemical messenger from one cell or group of cells to another. All multicellular organisms produce hormones.

ilium: In the pelvic area, the *ilium* is the lower front hip bone.

ligamentous: Relating to ligaments.

ligaments: Leathery strands of connective tissue between one bone and another.

lumbar: The five vertebrae between the ribs and the sacrum (L1 through L5).

lumbosacral: Refers to the region of the spine where the last lumbar vertebrae and the sacrum join (typically L5 and S1).

lumbosacral plexus: Formed where the nerves branch off the lumbar spine and form a bundle or group of nerves in the interior of the pelvis.

MRI: *Magnetic Resonance Imaging* is a test that produces clear images of the human body without using x-ray technology. Instead, a large magnet, radio waves, and a computer are used to generate images.

musculoskeletal: The structures of the body that include muscles, tendons, ligaments, bones, and joints.

myofascial release: Fingertip or other manipulation to loosen connective tissue.

nerve: Nerves conduct impulses from receptor organs to tissues and organs. A bundle or group of bundles of nerve fibers outside the central nervous system connects the brain and spinal cord with various parts of the body.

nerve entrapment: Phrase used to describe when a nerve is compressed or pinched in a narrow space, causing discomfort or pain and resulting in permanent or temporary injury.

nerve fiber: A small number of specialized cells transmitting impulses that convey information about sensations or cause movement.

nerve roots: Paired bundles of nerve fibers exiting the spinal cord between each two vertebrae; soon after leaving the spinal cord, nerve roots combine, and their fibers regroup into individual nerves.

orthopedist: A physician who specializes in problems of the form and function of bones, joints, and muscles.

osteoarthritis: A progressive degeneration of joints due to either normal or abnormal wear and tear.

patency: Refers to something anatomically that is open or unblocked.

pedicles: Two short thick processes that project backward, one on either side, from the upper part of the body at the junction of its posterior and lateral surfaces.

piriformis syndrome: The compression of the sciatic nerve by the piriformis muscle in the buttock.

proprioception: The sense of the relative position of neighboring parts of the body.

proprioceptors: A nerve receptor that responds to stimuli originating within the body itself, especially those responding to pressure, position, or stretch.

radicular: Refers to a pattern of pain, numbness, tingling, etc., from pressure on the nerve root.

radiculopathy: A compression or pinching of a spinal nerve root.

reflex: An involuntary movement brought about when nerves activate a muscle in response to a stimulus applied to a sensory nerve.

reflex sympathetic dystrophy: A painful imbalance arising from the automatic nervous system and usually affecting an arm or leg.

ruptured disc: See *herniated disc.*

sacroiliac joint derangement: A misalignment of the sacrum with respect to the iliac bones.

sacrum: A large central bone supporting the entire spinal column and wedged between the two sides of the pelvis.

S and L: Abbreviations for sacral and lumbar. Health care givers use these abbreviations (along with T for *thoracic* and C for *cervical*) to refer to specific spinal locations. They are usually associated with numbers that designate specific vertebrae. (For example, S3 is the third sacral vertebrae.) Both sacral and lumbar vertebrae are numbered from 1 to 5, thoracic vertebrae are numbered 1 to 12, and cervical vertebrae are numbered from 1 to 7.

sciatica: Pain or discomfort that travels down the buttock and leg in the pattern and path of the sciatic nerve, the body's largest nerve.

scoliosis: An abnormal curvature of the spine.

sign: A result of a diagnostic test; an objective indication of an injury or disease.

slipped disc: A misnomer. See *herniated disc.*

spasm: A painful, involuntary muscle contraction; the duration can be from minutes to months.

spinal stenosis: A narrowing of the lumbar or cervical spinal canal, which causes compression on nerve roots or the spinal cord.

spondylolisthesis: Forward slippage of a lumbar vertebra on the vertebrae below it, most often at the level between the fifth lumbar vertebrae and the first sacral vertebrae.

sprain: When fibers of a ligament or tendon are partially or completely torn.

subluxation: A minor misalignment of bones in a joint.

symmetrical: Occurring in the same place on both sides of the body.

symphysis: A fibrocartilaginous fusion between two bones.

symptom: Something you feel, such as a pain or tingling; a subjective indication of an injury or disease.

tendon: A strong leathery strand of tissue connecting a muscle to a bone or another muscle.

thixotropy: The property of certain gels of becoming less viscous when shaken or subjected to shearing forces and returning to the original viscosity upon standing.

thoracic: Referring to the part of the body enclosed by the ribs, including the spine from T1 through T12.

transthoracic: Across the *thorax*, the part of the body between the base of the neck and the diaphragm.

trimester: The nine months of pregnancy is divided into three trimesters. The *first trimester* is comprised of months one through three, the fourth through sixth months are the *second trimester*, and the final three months are the *third trimester*.

vascular: Having to do with arteries, veins, and the lymphatic system.

vertebrae: The bony segments of the spinal column.

visceral: The adjective *visceral* is used for anything pertaining to the internal organs.

INDEX